Medical History of Mankind

Medical History of Mankind

How Medicine is Changing Life on the Planet

Andrey Nabokov

To order additional copies of this book, contact:
Xlibris Corporation
0-800-644-6988
www.xlibrispublishing.co.uk
Orders@xlibrispublishing.co.uk
306333

Contents

Walls punched with the head.
Everything else—the only tools.

(Leszek Cumor)

Preface

Medicine as a serious branch of critically important knowledge, which entered into the everyday life of mankind, is not so old; it is just a few hundred years old. Judging by today's investments in it, the importance of medical knowledge and technology to governments and individuals is steadily growing. What will happen to medicine in the twenty-first century? What new capabilities will be there for mankind? In connection with this, how will the mankind change itself? Will it be healthier and how will it change the very concept of health in the future? What will happen with the health care system and why? Which relationships between medicine and health care system will there be in future? Will the tasks for health care providers be changed and how? Answers to these questions seem to me more important than the problem of future energy and space research, changes in climate, world food problems, and planetary reconciliation of inter-religious and ethnic hatred. It is not because I am not interested in these issues, but because in all of these issues the object is a human, and solutions should be found, namely, by the future mankind, whose image is forming precisely right now in the laboratories, institutes, and clinical departments, where people work in white coats. The only ones having the means and opportunity among all the scientists to change the 'measure of all things', that is the human being.

We live in a period of time when the most modern and new features and tools appear in human hands, power of which is incomparable to all that we have seen in the entire previous history. Many of these tools can be used to change the human as a biological object, his body and mind, and it only depends on him the way he applies them and for what they are used. It has been noted that the effects of many modern tools of mankind become clear only after the commencement of their real use.

The book you hold in your hands is an attempt to understand the medical history of mankind not only in a scientific and historical manner, with strictly selected facts and references to the historians, but also to see in the images that are visible as to how the attitude of mankind has changed towards himself and towards his body and its functions, as well as the changes in attitudes to illness and treatment and how medicine appeared in the past. Also, we will try to understand where medicine and health care industry are moving towards, the challenges they may face in the near future, and how this may impact the lives of mankind as a whole. The book will be of interest both to health professionals and to those who are interested in the development and future of medicine. Given the practical experience that absolutely everybody is well versed in the problems of modern medicine, we should expect that this book will have the widest audience.

Sincerely,
Author

Chapter 1

Medicine As a Selective Breeding of Biological Species

The phrase in the title of the first chapter looks a bit wild and unusual. And indeed, sitting in the waiting room before the doctor's office, who among us has thought about the question: what is the biological sense of the doctor's activity when he tries to repair our body? Every day on the planet, hundreds of thousands of doctors and nurses take several million of patients; the results of their work are the massive multidirectional changes in the patient's bodies. How does it affect the Homo sapiens with the general stream of time and does it affect at all? How do we imagine the purpose of this daily activity and what's its real product? Let's try to talk about it in this chapter.

1. A. What's the Goal of Medicine and How to Understand It

Health care is currently executing a great variety of tasks; the list of those tasks is slightly different in different countries, depending on many local factors. However, if we consider only medical problems, unlike general social problems, they are not just similar, but are identical for all countries, and it's not surprising, because they are aimed at the same object and solve the same objectives.

Tasks of a medical practitioner in our time, in general, are simple and clear (depending on specialisation), even for a lay person in the field of medicine, namely, as follows:

1. A doctor performs deliveries, i.e. supervises and directs (often literally) the process of bringing to life new individuals of species Homo sapiens. He also undertakes steps to ensure that the progeny may be born, even those that had been deprived of such opportunities without his help.
2. The physician identifies individuals who are sick, i.e. their bodies have deviations, and decides whether these deviations need to be corrected.
3. If it is decided that the deviations must be corrected, he tries to do it by using the methods accepted in the current stage of development of medical science.
4. If abnormalities exist, but current technology does not allow him to correct them, the physician takes measures to ensure the longest lifetime of the mentioned person.
5. If the current technologies do not provide ways to extend the life of the mentioned person, the physician takes steps to a more humane end of the patient's life.

That's what all the medical staff do on the planet while providing services to their patients. Read them again, if not hard.

Does this list of problems brings to mind something? If not, still let us remember our school textbook of biology.

> Selective breeding is a selective admission to breeding for animals, plants or other organisms in order to develop new varieties and breeds that have desirable qualities; it is the predecessor of modern plant and animal breeding. The basis of this breeding method is the variability of signs and their heritability.

> Selective breeding is one of the main methods of selection, which can be used both independently and in combination with other methods. (Wikipedia: http://ru.wikipedia.org)

I think that no one will deny that the Homo sapiens still has variability of signs and their heritability, otherwise it would not have been a part of the animal kingdom. Further, it should be recognised that, without a doubt, some part of the human population is constantly and methodically performing on the individuals of its own species the same actions that makes any breeder wonder how to preserve the breed of animals in an unfavourable environment, no matter how it is unpleasant to hear. If we express the meaning of this work in a word, it is likely that word would be 'counteraction'. What prevents a doctor and what's the purpose of the work?

All of the above actions of health workers en masse merge into a single act of will, which must be objective. It's clear that taken separately the modern physician cannot even conceive of such purposes as the performing of selective breeding of their patients for anything, but especially in the eugenic purposes. And, surely, doctors were not doing it in the past. So what is the purpose of medicine? First, let us agree on what is meant by the word 'medicine'. The generally accepted definition is as follows:

> Medicine is the applied science or practice of the diagnosis, treatment, and prevention of disease. It encompasses a variety of health care practices evolved to maintain and restore health by the prevention and treatment of illness in human beings. (Wikipedia: http://en.wikipedia.org)

This definition of medicine is very similar in their informational content to the phrase 'we treat patients so that they may be sound' and fascinating in its 'depth' and anthropocentrism. This definition emphasises that medicine is an activity aimed at the human body; for example, tens of thousands of veterinarians around the world (and not only them) are denied the right to be called health professionals. This definition was explicitly given by the person looking at the problem from within and because the initially inherent humanity does not think about simple questions, such as the following:

- What is the purpose of preserving and improving the health of people?
- What's the people's health? At what point, the natural processes in the human body should already be considered pathological?
- Who are these people and how to distinguish them from non-humans? Where is the exact limit of the human body?
- What is the role of humans on the planet and are they useful for our planet as a species?
- What if the health and growth of the number of people are hurting other species of this planet?
- Do we need to counteract natural processes in the population of people?

These questions themselves seem unnatural, inhumane; such questions probably should be asked from the non-humanoid aliens that overlook our planet and for whom humanity is just an abstraction (say, that our non-humanoid can think abstractly); one of the other 'isms' is a way to think in terms of interest of only one species.

So what is medicine in terms of a 'non-human', i.e. a being which is not humane by definition? What does practicing medicine at the macro level mean? Does it select individuals in accordance with certain criteria? Undoubtedly, this criterion is illness. That is, the first step is clearly negative selection, as healthy people are not much of interest to current physicians. What happens with selected people? Medicine leads them to the criterion of either 'not the norm, but treatable' or 'the impossibility of bringing to the norm'. Major efforts are directed to increase the life expectancy and increase the percentage of healthy progeny and their number. For these purposes, medicine uses specific technologies. Putting humans on par with all living beings on the planet and taking the situation into account, I propose the following definition of medicine and its goals:

> Medicine is a complex of knowledge and technologies based on those that allow the species to perform the selective breeding within its own species, having a purpose of countering the natural processes that inhibit the expansion of this species in the entire habitat available for him. It occurs at a certain stage of development of the species, when some of its individuals are able to affect the life expectancy and rate of reproduction in this and other species.

This extremely wide definition of medicine separated from the concept of 'human' raises a number of questions. So, therefore, can there be 'inhuman' medicine? Apparently so. Which are the examples? So far, the examples cannot be shown (let's set aside the green men and let's give the proof of its existence first),

15

because out of all terrestrial organisms only man has reached the stage in the development of knowledge where he has been able to systematically counteract natural processes of culling within his own population, thereby stimulating the expansion of his own species. Conversely, the fact is that the expansion of the Homo sapiens species prevents the development of other species on the planet and thus makes it impossible for other species to reach this stage. In general, we can also say that the fact that only this species has reached the stage of medicine over time makes this species the dominant on the planet. Further, it is appropriate to ask whether medicine only exists to spread mankind across the planet and explore new climatic zones and habitats. But what about humanity and helping our neighbours? The answer may lie in the fact that the concept of humanity and the tradition to help neighbours is a natural mechanism for the expansion of a species that lived in herds and were forced to invent ways of social communication. Medicine is just one of the next steps of this natural mechanism, designed as a scientific discipline and a set of practical technologies.

As we know from history, the profession of a doctor is one of the oldest professions; there is no nation, even the most ancient, that has not left us written sources that medical instruments were found in their cultural layers, as well as traces of surgery on bones and mummified remains, sometimes even quite complex. Moreover, we find traces of primitive interventions even in the bones of prehistoric ancestors who lived in caves. At the same time, for the modern great apes, even those that lived next to man, we cannot see the rudiments of medical activities (combing parasites from each other cannot be considered). Can we conclude that the man is a monkey in the stage of mastering medicine? It's doubtful. But, on the other hand, to deny such a conclusion would contradict what you see.

Species, which reached an evolutionary stage of the development of medicine could also use it for expansion (or vice versa—inhibition of development) of other species at will. Nobody will deny that pets that are close to humans for any purpose receive medical care from him and are in a state of controlled expansion. Most of the decorative animal species would not survive even for a few days in the wild. But in an artificial habitat created by man, they survive and produce healthy offspring only through the efforts of veterinarians. Even populations of many wild animals today are largely retaining their strength through the efforts of man who uses medical technology to support them in the struggle with their own intervention in the ecology of entire regions, water areas, and continents. As an example of human's inhibition of development of other species, we can recall the purposeful destruction of habitats of malarial mosquitoes, rodents, insects, fungi and pathogenic bacteria, and viruses.

When asked why a human uses medical technology in neighbouring species, we inevitably come to the conclusion that at some point of increasing the biological resources available for species the concept of humanism starts to include not only its own species but also those with whom he is emotionally connected, since they are constantly living beside him or available as 'canned meat' or as draft animals or as helpers in hunting, and today even as living home toys. The borderline of 'humanising' neighbouring biological species is very unstable and constantly moving in response to changes in the number of species, which is attracted to 'cooperation'. The most recent example is the changed attitude of mankind to horse, which from occupying the privileged position of being the main human friend in the early twentieth century has descended to the level of being just live sports equipment. It is also clear that as yet there is no requirement of humanistic treatment of earthworms or *Vibrio cholerae*, although their 'rights' in terms of law are validly distinguished from the 'rights' of cow or the favourite hunting dog.

The next section will attempt to trace why a certain stage of development of medicine and state is required in such a social phenomenon as the health care system.

1. B. When Does the Health Care System Appear and What's the Difference Between Medicine and Health Care System?

In the previous section, when a new definition of medicine was proposed, there was no indication that health workers carried out these goals consciously. You may ask, how it is possible to achieve some goals subconsciously? Did medical activity not reach its objectives until the very concept of 'species' and, really, even more, until the concept of 'selective breeding'? The fact is that human being became dominant on this planet long before understanding the biological meaning of his medical practice.

Indeed, an ancient person provided medical aid to his wounded fellow (albeit for money); he did just that and nothing more. Awareness of the fact that regular and methodical provision of medical care in the broadest sense can also be a long-term consequence for the whole tribe, and even for all mankind, came much later, when a person stopped presenting himself as a unique creation of God and put himself in line with all living beings on the planet and began to imagine long-term consequences of his medical efforts. It is set to the length of the causal relations that the public consciousness can accommodate. Only in the beginning of the nineteenth century did mankind learn to go to this level of generalisation and constructed logical chains of such length. In our case, a new understanding of the facts concerning human biology came only in the eighteenth- to nineteenth-century works of great naturalists and systematists of the living world (Carl Linnaeus, Peter Artedi, and Charles Darwin). Discovering the laws of heredity in the nineteenth century (Gregor Mendel) and deciphering the genetic code in the twentieth century (Francis Crick, James Watson, and Maurice Wilkins) radically changed the attitude of mankind to himself.

So when and why did a health system come into existence? It is logical to assume that physicians that were available encountered the problem (permanently or periodically repeated) that could not be resolved with scattered efforts. An example is mass circulation of patients with similar diagnoses in an epidemic or those injured in a major war (as a variant of traumatic epidemic). At this stage, the doctors' corporations came into existence, which had their own hierarchy distinct from the state and their own methods of solving problems. The first hardest lessons of this science were gained during an epidemic of plague and smallpox in the Middle Ages, which mowed the population of cities and entire countries. That was when monarchs and mayors first saw that the epidemic response required system actions to be performed on a specific plan.

In which society is the appearance of the health care system (further on referred to as HCS) most likely? We can say with some confidence that such a society has the following:

- a constant negative factor or a recurring threat to the population size; for example, being constantly engaged in war with its neighbours and having a steady stream of wounded.
- the only restriction to human resources so patients who need treatment have a value that society is compelled to return them 'in order'.
- already has an extensive medical practice and a number of experienced doctors.
- strict management and high degree of vertical organisation, which allows to set and achieve global goals.
- a proper density of population, in which one medic can serve many patients. That is, this indicator is a function of the mode of transportation to physicians and patients to each other, namely, the more the inaccessible care (patients slowly get to the doctor and vice versa), the more the need expressed to organise a system of care. We can say that the problem was low access to health care when walking was the first problem, for which the first primitive HCS began to come into existence.

It is not surprising that the first HCS was associated with military activities of humans, i.e. with the activity that produced the wounded. The more the armies became more regular and numerous, the more they needed a system of treating the wounded.

The first HCS to provide assistance, which we know originated in ancient Rome, had been organised by Claudius Galen, who worked as a doctor in the school of gladiators, first in Pergamum and later in Rome, where he was invited to take up the post of personal physician of Emperor Marcus Aurelius. He developed a system which had almost all the hallmarks of modern health care system and was required to oversee the preparation, training, and nutrition of gladiators, as well as treatment and care of them. Slave-gladiators were very expensive, and the emperor was interested in preserving and increasing their numbers, as well as their health as it affected their combat performance. Slaves were deliberately selected, provided with adequate food, coached by a special system that provided a mode for increasing combat capability, and given carefully customised armour and weapons. The wounded gladiators were treated by the best surgeon of that time—Claudius Galen of Pergamum and assistants trained by him, and the best postoperative care was provided. In addition, Galen did a lot of research and teaching work. It is likely that medical services for the gladiators were of even higher quality than that for ordinary legionaries and staff officers of the Roman Army. Of course, customers of such systems were only a few thousand people, but the fact remains that a system existed and carried out its tasks.

So what is the difference between just the medicine practiced by the individual (even qualified) doctors and the health care system? What are the signs of the forming health care system?

- The system is aware of the negative acting factor (threat). Keyword is 'aware'.

- The system takes various measures for survival of the population before the start of a negative factor. Keyword is 'before', so that is already predicted.
- The system is able to assess actions in terms of their effectiveness and chooses the best. Keywords are 'to assess measures'; that is, it does some kind of research, analysing the privies and present results.
- The system evaluates the doctors according to their individual performance and selects the best. Keywords are 'evaluates the doctors'; that is, it is able to assess the degree of qualification of doctors. The system at this stage already has a standard, which automatically becomes the best available doctor.
- The system unlike some practitioners has begun to move from the simple treatment to prevent morbidity in general because it has seen the cost-effectiveness of such an approach.
- The system supports itself (like any self-respecting system) and tries to preserve and develop its structure, so it carries *management*.

Thus, we can see that a group of doctors is not a health care system; yet it becomes the system when it is aware of its aims not at the level of individual customers, but for all potential patients at once, and has the means to follow these objectives. As awareness of the negative factors that threaten to reduce the population of a particular area and deprive the country of soldiers and workers, HCS developed various opposing measures that were initially in the city, in the region, and then in the whole country, forming, respectively, urban, regional, and national systems. With increase in the number of diverse problems, the specialisation of medical staff began.

With the complexity of the tasks that were set in front of physicians and their corporations, the following became clear:

- Doctors themselves could not be stakeholders for all tasks because tasks were too many, and they were intertwined and interacted with each other. It required a single *regulating point.*
- The further it was, the more it became clear that the credibility and authority of some doctors to perform the tasks was not enough. There were *efforts and support of the state* which were necessary.
- With the formulation and execution of tasks, it became clear that the knowledge and skills of the current generation of doctors were not enough. There was a need for *targeted training for health staff for carrying out the assigned tasks.*

Once the ruler of the country realised that the doctors' problems were because not only of their selfish reasons for obtaining a livelihood but also of vital interest to the ruler, the situation began to change. In all developed countries, the establishment of national health systems began almost simultaneously only at the end of the nineteenth century. Why so late? It seems to me that changing methods of warfare had played a role. Battles had become so widespread, and the affected patients and wounded were so much that the belligerents (almost all developed countries in all continents were fighting till the end of the nineteenth century) were seriously preoccupied with the conservation of their human resources. One way or another, the entire population was involved in war, not just the vassals of the kings and mercenaries.

How should the health care system be defined? The classical definition is as follows:

> A health system [. . .] is the organization of people, institutions, and resources to deliver health care services to meet the health needs of target populations. (From Wikipedia: http://en.wikipedia.org)

With this definition, we can conclude that health care is a *function of the whole society*, as it only affords to cover a range of activities varying over properties and to the extent that they relate to the public health. Medicine itself is referred to in the definition among other measures, and now it is clear that modern health care system does not consist of medical staff only, as many people think. Now, let's try to give this definition a biological sense in terms of the more general goals:

> Health care is a way to organise life within the species, which aims to ensure its survival in the given environment and to provide the development in accordance with certain goals that used medicine as instrument, as well as all social institutions that were developed in a given society.

From this definition, it follows:

Health care is, namely, a *way of organising life*, because there is no aspect of life of the individual or society as a whole that in some way does not affect the health system. Moreover, if such a side of life is found, it only indicates lack of development of the given HCS or dropping this individual out from the society.

Health care should be *in line with those objectives, which the species set for itself*. Problems can be formulated in a fuzzy form (depending on the logic of thinking and political structure of a particular society). It is important to emphasise that the HCS does not set the tasks for itself. If the given species is in civilisation impasse, the public health does not know itself where and why it has to move.

Health care *uses all the social institutions of the given society*: medicine itself, science, religion, family, army, law, culture, and politics (as a control method). Whatever the means of social communication that has not been invented by this society, they will all be included in the most important task—the preservation and development of biological species, which is assigned to the HCS.

In the next section, we try to understand at what stage are the disparate actions of individual doctors merged together and begin to affect the development of population.

1. C. Who Is the Breeder:
Doctor or Health Care System?

Admittedly, the question posed in the heading is far too much for a modern physician. However, if we trace the consequences of actions of individual physicians at different historical stages and then compare them with those of the modern health care system, then the question becomes a practical concern. Once we have defined medicine as a kind of 'machine' for the implementation of selective breeding within a species according to their objectives, then a positive answer suggests itself. However, the answer is not so easy.

The doctor who worked in the stage before appearing the HCS decided how many and which patients to treat and in which territory to treat them. He was, if I may say so, a 'freelancer'. In some ancient nations, where the art of healing had come from outside, doctors initially were slaves captured from the more civilised nations. In particular, every wealthy Roman citizen sought to acquire a slave-medic (*servus medicus*), usually of Greek origin. This slave-medic treated his master and his family. The value of such a slave gradually increased, and after a certain time, the owners let them free to earn for a fee. Legally, these doctors or freed men remained dependent on the slaveholders, and the Roman society treated them with some disdain for a long time. But the society inevitably came to the conclusion that the doctor when free was much more valuable than as a servant.

The possibility of a patient to see a doctor was determined by many factors, not least of which was his financial viability. The government generally did not address the issues of relationships between doctor and patient, believing it to be their own business. Medical service in those days was not fundamentally different from any other sales transaction.

As a result, citizens who could ask for help from such a 'freelance' doctor had to meet certain requirements:

- *Be able to pay for doctor's services*—Selection on social grounds, i.e. to be successful. However, it should be remembered that social success in those days was usually hereditary, for the treatment of slaves was paid by the master.
- *Have the physical ability to go to the doctor* or to pay his way in amount exceeding the profits lost from the time of the visit—i.e. the selection of the place of residence (a physician was not in each locality) and again on social grounds. With the growing affluent population in the area, doctors 'settled' in the same place, but where the population was small it was the poor itinerant doctors who appeared from time to time.
- *Have the disease the treatment of which could be done by a doctor*—There was not a doctor for every patient in those days, and not every illness or injury was then considered a curable problem. That is, it was selection by pathology type.
- *Not be an outcast in the given society*—In some societies, there were people with whom the doctor would never make a deal even if they had money. Such contacts were simply forbidden (usually on religious or national grounds). That is, there was a selection based on ethnic or religious grounds.
- *Be a relative of the doctor*—for good reasons.

Adding all the factors together, we can see that during prolonged (two to three generations) medical activities in the human population of the area social and demographic changes gradually accumulated, which can be briefly described as follows:

- *Mortality of the financially secured class (adult and child) decreased*, while that of the poor one was not changed. A special effect was a reduction in infant mortality in wealthy families. It is clear that the demographic imbalance accumulated so slowly that to notice it then would be very doubtful, even using modern statistical methods, because sampling would be very small. Thus, the presence of a competent physician in the territory was a factor to increase the overall population in the area, and namely, the wealthy population percentage increased. The territory became richer in its own eyes.

- *Decreased deadweight loss of command* during warfare for those armies which have more skilled doctors. It was understood to be so even in ancient times. In support of it there is a line by Homer: 'Many warriors is a skilled healer.' Since ancient times, the doctor was the man who along with a talented commander could really reduce the loss of all sorts in the hostilities. Gradually, aid extended to all ordinary soldiers.

- *Pathology in the eyes of the population was divided* into the one for which it made sense to call the doctor and that when it was useless (or even prohibited because of religious issues). The population was getting used to interacting with the doctors, and it had even taken over the simplest skills of self- and mutual aid. The more the patients that could use the services of a doctor, the more the population became literate in the medical sense; firstly, the closed knowledge gradually spread wider and wider. It could also include a wide dissemination of knowledge about primitive pharmacology and herbal medicine in all nations.

- *Percentage of outcasts* (religiously or culturally isolated communities, which the local doctors did not treat) *slowly lagged* behind in growth due to natural mortality. An exception occurred in cases where they had their own doctors.

- *Children (and family in general) of physicians had a much greater chance of survival* and longer life (in this case, their social success or religious and cultural isolation did not matter). Thus, physicians were the socio-privileged group (along with the elite); they had someone to pass on their skills. The number of their descendants grew, and this process was much less dependent on the overall mortality in the given territory. There were closed medical school clans, consisting of physicians' immediate relatives and their students.

Of particular importance was the emergence of physicians who provided care to children and women in maternity care, while doctors were beginning to directly affect the rate of reproduction in the current population or rather among the elite and middle class. The more pronounced the tendency among doctors to accompany their patients throughout their lives, the greater the impact of the services of physicians on the population size in general.

On summarising, we can say that in a society where a physician or a group of physicians is acting for a long time, natural processes of changing the size and quality of the population begin to become distorted and are replaced by artificial ones. The specific pattern of these processes may differ depending on whether it is because of the public health system already present or the group of doctors simply performing tasks set for themselves and their customers. As soon as the HCS appeared, which by definition had a goal, all social, biological, demographic, political, and economic processes in the population gradually changed to achieve these goals. Thus, we can conclude that the *conscious breeder in society is the health care system* rather than individual physicians.

1. D. The Minimal Functional Unit of the Health Care System

In studying any health system that is useful to mentally take it apart into small elements and see how they interact, the question is to what smallest details can the modern health care system (hereinafter HCS) be disassembled that this unit is still worked as the system on a comparable scale? In other words, where's the lower limit of scaling? As stated above, HCS 'from birth' characterised by the fact that it is aware of development goals, forecasts, estimates the measures taken and their performers by the degree of efficiency, and supports itself on the level of the given tasks. Of what the simplest HCS at a minimum level of functionality can consist of?

It is clear in this unit at least 'an object of care', namely patient, must be present, otherwise everything else is meaningless. Is it enough for *one* patient to perform the above functions? Judging health, we must acknowledge that the answer is no, because the lifetime of such a system would be equal to the lifetime of the patient, then the system would die due to lack of 'customers', not to mention any development. To prevent the system's death and to allow it to grow, it is necessary to cause next-generation 'customers', i.e. patients should multiply. Thus, we concluded that the minimum number of patients for the health care system are two opposite sex subjects who would be able to reproduce. We used to call this a family, without regard for possible legal niceties.

Next question: Is it enough for only *one* doctor to perform all the functions of HCS in relation to the minimum client (family)? We can imagine the doctor to be having a very broad profile of specialisation, who monitors the health of the entrusted family and its progeny and provides therapeutic activities when needed. Can we assume this is the HCS? I think not, because our general physician should appear from somewhere; someone has to teach him diagnose and treat, to supply him with the concepts of 'healthy' and 'unhealthy', 'benefit' and 'harm'. In this case, I'm not even talking about the technical equipment for the diagnostic and treatment process because medicine began with herbal medicine and regime so that the technique is still left in peace. So we come to the conclusion that the doctor (conventionally called 'performer' because HCS, as we found in the previous sections, consists not just of doctors) cannot appear from 'nowhere'; as well as within our system, he must be prepared practically and theoretically and get it 'outside'. The appropriate technologies he used must be developed by someone and his objectives should be explained by someone.

Thus, we can see that there should be another element of the system which puts together the global problems of health and prepares technologies and personnel for these tasks. We conventionally call him 'planner'. The same planner keeps track of the performance of the 'executive' as a whole, and over time, it corrects his tasks, predicts the situation, and creates and sustains the production of appropriate treatment and diagnostic tools, as well as the appropriate legal framework.

Does our mini-system need someone else to perform its functions at this level? I have not found so. Thus, our minimal cell of HCS consists of (a) a family, as a minimum client, (b) a prepared physician-executive, and (c) a planner of tasks and supervisor of the results. Our system is still 'hanging in the air'; yet it's out of economics, politics and the legal field, moral imperatives, and other attributes of human society.

By placing our mini system in the economic environment, we immediately realise that what is *beneficial* to the planner was one for all mini systems, because this work is the same (or nearly identical) for all cells, so it can pay once for all. Putting it in the political environment (as a medium of effective management of society), we see that is advantageous to have *one* planner, as his managerial functions are just the same for all cells in the system. Placing our cell in a legal field (as a system of written moral imperatives adopted in a given society), we see again that it is advantageous to have *one* common planner, as this will automatically provide the same legal support for all disputed cases arising in the client's health care by executives and transfer of successful results achieved to the neighbouring cells. By placing our system in a cultural and scientific environment, we see that it is *beneficial* to have *one* common planner, as this provides the centralised and standard preparation of all executives by the same methodology.

Thus, we can see that in real modern society, the cells of the health care system, barely born, immediately 'socialise' their planners, and not because they love to march in formation, but because this community is generally *cheaper* for the end customers, which support all participants of our system. That is the real configuration of the HCS cell determined by considerations of gain, namely, economic demands. We come into the picture when the HCS has the *one* global planner that outlines the tasks and measures for the survival of the species in the given habitat, a number of executives trained by a planner, and all the rest are the clients of the system. Move on.

In the next section, we'll try to understand if the object of care in the HCS changes over time, and if so, what does it depend on?

1. E. What's the General Direction of the Human Evolution?

In this issue, for the present we are interested namely in the biological component because the evolution of spiritual and social life of mankind is a very individual issue and because other professionals are engaged in this. So the simple question is: How was a human biologically changed for the entire time of observation?

Anthropologists insist that over the past several thousand years human as a biological object did not change; that is, a creature that anthropologists have called Cro-Magnon still exists. On the other hand, they argue that a human has ceased to evolve, unlike all other species on Earth, meaning it is contrary to evolutionary theory that has not yet been disproved. How can we ignore the evolution of man?

Well, firstly, mankind over time was divided into races and become a bit 'higher' due to the phenomenon of acceleration. Secondly, differences in the diets of isolated peoples have led to minor differences in the proportions of digestive juices and enzymes in different nations, the length of their intestines, as well as differences in response to some natural poisons and medicines. In closed ethnic groups, consistently inherited diseases observed with different frequency then were found in the rest of the mankind. Can we already consider this as the sign of human evolution?

I think no; the system simply accumulates diversity that is useless in this situation. With regard to races, they just do not have time to develop to the extent of the fundamental differences when people of different races can already be regarded as separate species (or at least subspecies) of Homo sapiens. Already it is clear that globalisation is rapidly mixing all the races, after which the racial differences will disappear as well as the small differences in the physiologies of digestion.

Thirdly, speaking about the human evolution, they speak, of course, not about the evolution of individuals, but about the evolution of a big enough group of them, which can be observed in the same conditions. Even Darwin pointed out that 'some individuals do not evolve, but their community—the population' do.

So what is the evolutionary process for human?

The fact that the human gradually became higher and, thus, became more and more a large mammal, I think, was underestimated in the literature. In this case, each extra centimetre of average height of mankind could make a difference. In the work of the famous anthropologist Robert Foley, *Another Unique Species: Patterns of Human Evolutionary Ecology* some evolutionary implications of enlargement of the body size of mammals and, in particular, the hominids were listed:

1. Increasing the size of the body can expand the food niche of animals. Since the increase in the size of animals is accompanied by a slower growth of their energy needs, the larger animals need less energy daily per mass unit.
2. Increasing the size of animals is accompanied by enlargement of the territory in which they move in search of food throughout the year (individual plots) or the day.
3. Increased body size is accompanied by increased mobility of animals.
4. Increased body size was accompanied by changes in relations of predator and prey. Opportunities of predator limited by dimensions of the prey he can catch.
5. Increased body size was accompanied by increased efficiency of thermoregulation (decreased cooling efficiency of the organism or increased insulation and ability to retain the heat). Increasing the size of the body improves the adaptation to the cold habitats and obstructs the adaptation to hot ones.

6. Increase in the size of the body was usually accompanied by an increase in the life expectancy.
7. Increase in the body size was associated with the slowing reproduction. Extending the all life stages, including pregnancy and period of postnatal development. This means that the 'value' of each baby to the population increases. Natural selection perpetuates the adaptive strategies that enhance the survival of their offspring.
8. Increase in the size of the body can be accompanied by increased social relations between animals. Selection in large mammals' populations occurs in the ability to recognise relatives and in their ability to behave with relatives in another way than with non-relatives. Group selection, altruism, and cooperation among large mammals distributed more widely than among the small ones.
9. Increase in the size of mammals may be accompanied by increase in the size of the brain. It is possible that this factor correlates with the duration of life of the animal and the accumulation of information about past periods as well as the social relationships in the population.

After reading all the items of evolutionary consequences of body enlargement, you are probably surprised to see how exactly they fit into the human representation of its own evolution. Thus, we can assume that the increase in the average height of human in the last few tens of thousands years for a few tens of centimetres had and continues to have implications for human evolution, and it changes not so much our anatomy, but our *behaviour*.

I believe that the evolution of Cro-Magnon is moving into another non-biological form because of the fact that he did not need to biologically compete more with anyone on the planet. Now the evolutionary process occurs in relations of human population with its environment. Evolution, as we know from the textbooks, happens under external pressure. A lot of factors can pressurise, but the most that can pressurise are the factors of the diet structure, as well as temperature, light, radiation, humidity, etc. Pressure can be performed also by competing with neighbouring species. If the species does not exert pressure, its biological evolution slows to a complete invisibility; such a situation happened with crocodiles, turtles, cockroaches, sharks. They have not changed for tens of millions of years, because their way of interacting with the external environment has not changed; that is, their ecological niche is stable. According to anthropologist Robert Foley, 'evolution is the process of solving problems', respectively: If the species have no problem, there is no evolution.

Man is the only species on the planet, which over time has separated its breed from the medium more and more and is increasingly becoming the creator of its own ecological niche. Caveman who would be dressed in animal skins thus has created the shell for himself, which separated him from the temperature vagaries of nature and created his first 'handmade' niche which the nature could not provide for him or rather could. But humans did not wait until hair could be acquired in a natural way in the cold climate of the next glaciation and borrowed the ready-to-use fur from animals. That is, people artificially accelerated the evolution in the desired destination. Since then, human consistently surrounded himself with shells, enclosing his own species one on top of another, like onions. A weapon was the shell against the competing predators. House and hearth were the shells that separated human from the weather in general, a kind of 'clothing for the whole family'. Then agriculture and animal husbandry came as shells which allowed them to be not dependent on natural harvests of some edible plant species and the abundance of some animals in the area. Then cities appeared as a shell that allowed a group of people to be separated from the natural habitat in general and live in an artificial environment. Forced to live in crowded cities because of the changed mode of production, they met the threat which wasn't previously familiar to them and the enemy they had not noticed before—epidemics that ravaged the entire countries. Against this new enemy, the old shells did not work. There was a need of a new type of shell: Not being able to destroy the enemy, to survive human was first forced to change himself. It was the vaccination against infectious diseases which fulfilled the role of another shell that separated man from the pathogenic microorganisms (non-pathogenic flora continued to exist within a human organism, but this wasn't known in those days).

Looking at modern man, we can see that the number of shells that he surrounds himself with are transformed into quality, which has decisively changed the way our species interact with the environment. People are increasingly not taking food, but energy for food production from the external environment. Human has fewer and fewer needs for different kinds of 'things' from his planet for production, but more and more energy to produce all these 'things'. Human is increasingly becoming a planetary phenomenon which is separated from his planet, just like we exist separately from the bricks that are used to build our house. Thus, human evolution has become artificial since humans have the opportunity to guide the evolution of their own species in the desired direction. In particular, we are able to go beyond the previously established 'old' shells by creating new, much wider ones, thereby increasing the degree of our evolutionary freedom. So far, the 'evolutionary space' of our species is limited in size with capability of land on our planet, but it is clear already that this barrier is very temporary. Modern mankind is gradually disabling the 'driving belts' of evolution, i.e. those feedbacks with which the planet could affect the species and square it 'for itself'. Temperature, water, and food dependence of humans have almost disappeared; at least, people believe that if there are no global and drastic changes in water and climatic balance of the planet and, consequently, in the flora and fauna, nothing serious is threatened from this side. What remain are solar radiation, atmospheric pressure, and its composition, which are still globally influencing the species of Homo sapiens, as well as the majority of the inhabitants of the planet.

All these general considerations help us to understand the place of the health system among all these shells, making the species of Homo sapiens independent from their natural habitat, which as we have already identified is nothing else but *the way to organise the life* of the species that want to achieve certain goals. First of all, HCS is the shell that protects a human from *evolutionary dangerous flaws* in the design of his own body. HCS allows the following:

1. Dramatically reduces the natural mortality from some diseases and injuries.
2. Reduces the mortality from some (ideally, all) infectious diseases.
3. Generally prevents epidemics of infectious diseases, changing the body of humans in a way that pathogenic flora does not harm it (i.e. either not in contact with humans or ceases to be pathogenic to him).
4. Alters the functional characteristics of the natural organs and tissues of the human body.
5. Replaces the human organs and tissues that are out of order with artificial ones.
6. Creates entirely new organs and tissues for functions that previously were not required, for example, to develop new habitats or for digesting new types of food.
7. Lengthens the average lifetime of the individual to the highest possible limits, including the preservation of all kinds of activity.
8. Provides practical *in vitro* fertilisation without both parents.

All of these tasks except, perhaps, fifth and sixth points have already begun to be resolved. That is, summing up, we can say that at the moment mankind is learning the skills of controlled artificial evolution, allowing him to be completely separate from the processes taking place on his planet and breaking the link with its flora and fauna.

To become a completely artificially evolving being, humans will need the following:

- eliminate or neutralise all natural enemies and competitors on the planet, including microorganisms,
- learn how the number of people and sex composition of the population can be fully controlled,
- eliminate the phenomenon of disability,
- learn to create new or modify old organs and tissues to meet the new needs and functions of the human body,
- develop new habitats: ocean and upper atmosphere,
- learn how to create habitats with artificial insolation (lighting), pressure, and composition of atmosphere,
- simplify or significantly standardise the nutrition process to cease the dependence on the distribution areas of cereals on the planet and not exclude the appearance of elements of external digestion in one form or another.

Side effects in this way will be the following:

- *Prolongation of the active life of the individual to the maximum possible and/or desirable limits*: As a consequence, the significant ageing of the population of the planet, in fact, changed the very concept of 'old age'. For example, about 300 years ago, people at 60 years was regarded as almost a long-living person, but now this is a common thing, and moreover, we say that a man who is dead at 50 years has 'had died young'. If the trend continues in the late twenty-first century, man at 90 years would be considered as 'not old yet'.

- *Significant reduction in the number of species on the planet*: Domesticated or 'decorative' species have survived while wild species have drastically reduced in number and diversity. The same thing happens with the plant world.
- Artificial ways of regulating the sex structure of the population will lead to *distortions in the ratio of men and women in different parts of the world*, and it may produce male and female demographic 'waves' which would overlap in different regions in the most unpredictable ways.
- *The process of eating will be unified*: Namely, it may be reduced to receiving the standard feed mixtures overdosed with calories. The ancient process of 'meal', i.e. eating natural organic food, will be the privilege of the elite.
- *Significant allergisation of population.* This will lead to appearing the closed antigen-free residential zones where people will live, but an attempt to go out of which may be very dangerous because of threat of anaphylactic shock.
- Creation of artificial organs and tissues for new functions of the human body could lead to *fashioning the structure of the body, certain features, and their combinations*. Humanity has become much more diverse, for now anatomically.
- *Increase in the number of population in different countries will cease to be an indicator of development.* There will be gradual loss of institutions such as citizenship. The population in developed countries will be 'common'.

In the next section, we will see which factors would cause the artificial evolution of humans and what relation would the health care system have to this.

1. F. Does the Mankind Be Divided Apart?

The question posed in the heading can be answered in different ways. The main difference between them is on what grounds does it make sense to make the division? In the past, the population of species Homo sapiens was divided into groups on the basis of the following criteria:

- Those who were able to maintain fire and those who could not.
- Those who were capable of articulating speech and those who were not capable of such.
- Those who were able to make clothes and those who could not.

After some time, the criteria for dividing were slightly changed:

- Those who knew written language and those who did not.
- Those who knew how to make iron tools and those who did not know.
- Those who had their own state and those who did not have.

Each century brought new signs by which mankind could be divided. Sometimes these signs were visible at once, and sometimes these symptoms became apparent after some time, even for their descendants. With this division, the presence of these signs was considered as progress and a lack thereof was considered moving backwards. The disadvantage of such a division was its artificiality and temporality, because the signs for the division always were knowledge and skills of the human. Signs of separation which were considered essential in one century invoked a smile in the next century. The only signs that a person could not change were his race and gender.

Nowadays, no one is trying to divide mankind with such transient signs. Recognition of racial differences does not give anything as this visible sign has no effect on what can be considered as essential features in our time. In addition, the races will become more and more mixed in the process of globalisation. What do we believe are essential signs right now? The average lifespan of mankind is constantly growing, and it was noticed long ago. Recent studies show that they do not just grow, but grow exponentially. Here are the data presented by Ray Kurzweil (The Singularity Summit at Stanford, 2006):

Table 1. Increase in average life expectancy

Period of history	Life expectancy (years)
Cro-Magnon (30,000-25,000 years ago)	18
Ancient Egypt (3,000 years ago)	25
1400, Europe	30
1800, Europe and the United States	37
1900, USA	48
2002, USA	78

This table shows the fact that the increase in the average lifespan from 18 to 25 years (increment of 7) took about 20,000 years. But for the next increment of 30 years (from 48 to 78 years) has taken a total of 100 years, although this figure was calculated for a single country. If we were to plot this growth, it is clear that mankind has entered a period of almost vertical rise in life expectancy; that is, in the next 10-20 years, humans will reach the times increasing in terms of their lives. But note that we are talking about the average life expectancy. Different individuals in different countries will have dramatically different lifespans.

Apparently, an essential sign of separation in our time can be considered the *average life expectancy* (ALE) of an individual. Life expectancy at birth is the average number of years that a newborn infant would have lived under the condition that at each age the conditions in life remain as they were for the corresponding age group in the year of his birth. This sign is almost independent of the knowledge and skills of the individual, but depends on the rather ambiguous concepts, such as healthy food, comfortable living environment, ecological environment, efficient medical care, lack of hereditary diseases, education, diet preferences, mental constitution and ability to handle stress, regular exercise and lifestyle. All these features are inherent in individuals belonging to the society at a certain stage of development without the rigid dependency on the nationality or race as well as state boundaries. After relocating the person into another society that is very different from the characteristics of the original one, the life expectancy will change smoothly up or down, but the real value of ALE will no longer be related to it.

Indicative data from U.S. studies to the reduction in ALE that is dependent on certain factors are listed in Table 2.

Table 2. Reduction in average life expectancy (ALE) that is dependent on certain factors

The reason for risk in reducing the life expectancy	Reduction in ALE, days
Living below the poverty line	3,500
Is a man (not a woman)	2,800
Smoking (one pack of cigarettes per day)	2,300
Cardiovascular disease	2,100
Overweight	900
Inadequate medical service	550
Alcohol	230

As can be seen from this table, ALE is a very integral index, and the first three principal factors include income, gender, and smoking factors. Other smaller factors can be combined under the symbolic flag of 'medical care'.

Another sign of the division of mankind, in my opinion, is the *degree of adaptability of the individual*. Psychologists talk about the different ability to withstand stress; teachers talk about the different degree of learning. Doctors also have an opinion about this, and they talk about stability and elasticity of the nervous system and say a lot of buzzwords in this regard. However, we cannot deny that people differ markedly in their ability to perceive the new, to adapt to it and to live in it. The future comes more and more faster, and the person who can match him has a much greater chance of survival. There is no evidence that this sign depends on the racial-ethnic factor, but there is evidence that it depends on the next sign.

Age: It is difficult to imagine the more transient and changing sign. Indeed, in past centuries, age was only about the degree of social trust and respect for the man. In traditional societies, the older the person was, the more he was respected and considered valuable and closer to the elite. There was no difference in the lifestyles of young and old persons. Nowadays, the world is constantly accelerating, and there is a significant difference in lifestyles of different generations and it affects both ALE and the degree of adaptability, because reality forces the young people to live in a style of continuous changes and provides a kind of selection for better adaptability. And adaptability is not required as a temporary sign for a young person, but as a permanent and lifelong attribute. Thus, the very high adaptability and lifelong learning ability have the potential to gain a foothold as a sign of species for Homo sapiens.

The structure of the body: Here we're not talking about the differences in growth and tendency to be overweight in certain nations. The fact is that there has been a distinct trend for countries with advanced medicine and that some of the citizens have serious differences in the structure and functions of the body. The number and range of such differences is gradually increasing, among which are the following:

- Massive bypass surgery of coronary arteries in the elderly population
- Numerous installations of the heart valves and pacemakers
- Numerous installation of endoprosthesis (mainly knee and hip) of large joints
- Implantable hearing devices and artificial lenses
- Implantable orthopaedic fixators in the bones (plates, screws, artificial ligaments, etc.)
- Numerous dental implantable devices.

It is clear that such a massive 'modernisation' of citizens' bodies not only has demographic consequences (in terms of lengthening the life expectancy) but also has economic consequences. The 'streamlined' population continues to work actively even after formally retiring and generates an additional social product, which gives the community a considerable economic advantage. These differences in the structure and functions of the body can and will have consequences for society:

- Once *upgraded, the body cannot be reduced to its initial look.* It's impossible to simply remove without loss a coronary bypass from artery, blood vessel prosthesis, or artificial heart valve as well as joint endoprosthesis. That is, such changes are lifelong, and the percentage of such population in developed countries is growing.
- However, a *streamlined body is relatively easily subjected to further modernisation*, such that a heart valve can be replaced by a more modern and reliable one, the revision joint arthroplasty can be accomplished as well

as the pacemaker may be replaced, etc. In other words, modernisation pulls the other upgrades more progressively and profoundly. The process of modernisation of the human body becomes continuous, and sooner or later, it will also include the nervous system. Prostheses of organs of senses are the first prerequisites for this.

- Gradually an *entire new branch of industry has appeared*, which has developed and established the devices for modernisation inside the human body. Thus, the 'modernisation' of people as a breakthrough of medical technology becomes a routine business. This business soon can become so much routine that it will begin to engage the state.

- Indications of the body's 'modernisation' are continuously increasing and the contingent of such people will *get younger* all the time. Once these people become the majority, this fact will be reflected in the legislation.

- *Way of life and lifestyle of* 'modernised' *people gradually acquire new capabilities*, unattainable for people of their age. Simultaneously, lifestyle restrictions occur, which are related with permanently taking drugs, the influence of electromagnetic fields as well as aggressive environments. That is, the lifestyle of such people is changing.

Clearly, all these upgrades are lifelong, but not heritable. But they do not need to be inherited by the creature which is preparing for artificial evolution. As we refine the process of installing such devices, the routine manipulation perceived as something exceptional ceases and becomes an indispensable attribute of every person to achieve some 'age of modernisation', a sort of routine inspection and maintenance of needs and capacities of the body. Occupational differences in the structure of the body also become possible.

Thus, adding all these essential signs, which may divide mankind, we can obtain the following situation:

- On the one hand, part of the population lives significantly longer (the ALE is higher) than the other and thus accumulates more individual and systematic knowledge that may be passed to the next generation in ready-to-use form. *The collective experience of such a long-living society is immeasurably greater* than the short-living one.

- On the other hand, the long-living part of mankind not only lives longer but also differently. Additional activity of the 'streamlined' population leads to a lot more consumers for goods and services, which is essential for the growth of specific markets in the areas densely populated by such people. *Long-living population gradually develops a specific style of life peculiar only to them.* On the other hand, there is a short-living population for which this style of life is not only inconvenient and incomprehensible but also even biologically inacceptable in some cases.

- High level of ALE in conjunction with a high degree of adaptation and learning capabilities provides an explosive mixture: The elderly 'streamlined' people cease to be an example of conservatism and the 'good old days'; instead they are actively involved in the modern pilot studies and projects. They are always willing to try and experiment and are prepared to teach others. On the other hand, there are the *short-living old population* with a low degree of adaptation and senile bodies, which *fall out of the process of accelerating technological progress* and remain in the sidelines.

Thus, we see the division of mankind on the basis of a set of attributes that lead to the gradual formation of two branches:

Long-living mankind with a high degree of readiness for the new, the desire for changes, and a 'milestone-modernised' body.

Short-living mankind with a low degree of readiness for the new, fear of changes, and a sick, senile body.

Separation will be enhanced by the fact that these two halves will not need each other and will not treat each other as competitors. The style of life, the goals, and vital needs, including the biological ones after some time, will be so different that they scatter into different ecological niches and will need different things, both in terms of spiritual and physiological needs. One-way transfer between the branches will be possible: The representatives of a short-living branch can join the long-living branch, but not vice versa. It is clear that the more younger the age that this transfer is made, the more the benefits will be obtained.

Are there any first signs of division of mankind in the branches? Here, of course, we can recall that the average resident of Andorra has lived almost three times longer than the average resident of Mozambique or Botswana (see Table 3, CIA 2003). Of course, if a child from Botswana will be moved to Japan and integrated into the new society, then he is likely to live there much longer than his peers at home, but he will live still less than the average Japanese native of the same age group. That is, some factors that we carry in ourselves, inside our own bodies, come into play here. At the common level, this is called 'inheritance'. As soon as we recognise it, we should also automatically recognise the inhomogeneity of the present mankind which is manifested in varying degrees of longevity, and this inhomogeneity will be inherited as an internal factor, unlike the external technological factors.

Table 3. Average life expectancy (ALE) in some countries of the world*

#	Country	ALE	Region
1	Andorra	83.49	Europe
2	San Marino	81.43	Europe
3	Japan	80.93	Asia
. . .			
115	Honduras	66.65	North America
116	Ukraine	66.50	Europe
117	Sao Tome and Principe	66.28	Africa
. . .			
190	Zambia	35.25	Africa
191	Botswana	32.26	Africa
192	Mozambique	31.30	Africa
Note: According to CIA (July 2003).			

Does this fact mean that there is already a fundamental difference in the inhabitants of Botswana and Japan? If we make a thought experiment and equalise these two countries socially and technologically, retaining such parity during several generations, will they not be equal in the average life expectancy? That is to say, the technological advantage of some society is constantly and gradually accumulating in the bodies of its inhabitants, and these differences start to descend. The speed of these changes seems dependent on the openness of a society, including the degree of influx of fresh genetic material from 'outside'.

The same is true for other signs of separation: willingness to changes and lifestyle. Lifestyles of Central African villages and modern Tokyo or New York are like two different planets, and the differences are not only in transportation and consumer electronics. These differences relate to all aspects of life from birth to death, including the physiological aspects (childbirth, breastfeeding, food and drinks, sending natural needs, work, illness, death). Willingness to change in the average resident of Japan, who has experienced in his lifetime several periods, several technological revolutions, as well as countless changes in fashion, and who saw his great-grandchildren and played strange electronic games with them, is many times greater than the willingness to change and adaptability of a resident of equatorial Africa, who has never left his native village in his entire thirty-year life. Note that I do not use the concepts of 'better' or 'worse' and 'high' or 'low'. I just want to say that these people are different.

Sharp (almost three times!) differences in the average lifespan will inevitably change the nature of man as a 'cultural animal'. The longer the person lives, the greater the experience he accumulates and can transmit to their descendants as a cultural heritage. Thus, the two processes reinforce each other: Longevity stimulates the overall number and diversity of culture transmitted to descendants, and culture (including science) encourages research to lengthen the lifespan. Nonlinear mutual acceleration of these processes is occurring within our sight.

Summary of the First Chapter

So let's try to summarise the contents of the first chapter. It was argued that the conventional definition of medicine from the encyclopaedia gave us almost nothing to understand human needs in health care and its role in the evolution of species. A *new definition of medicine* was given:

> *Medicine* is a complex of knowledge and technologies. Based on them, the species are allowed to perform the selective breeding within its own species, having the purpose of countering the natural processes that inhibit the expansion of this species in the entire habitat available for the species. It occurs at a certain stage of the development of the species, when some of its individuals are able to affect the life expectancy and rate of reproduction in this and other species.

This definition provides an understanding of medicine as a social mechanism for artificial selection in the interests of a particular species. We came to the conclusion that the conscious breeder in the society is HCS, not the individual doctors.

We also saw that a group of doctors are not the health care system; but the group becomes system when there is awareness of its purpose not only at the level of individual patients but also all potential patients and has the means to follow these purposes.

A *new definition of health care* was given, namely:

> *Health care* is a way to organise life within the species, which aims to ensure its survival in the given environment and to provide the development in accordance with certain goals that used medicine as instruments, as well as all social institutions that were developed in a given society.

We understand that the minimum cell of the health system consists of (a) a family, as a minimum client, (b) the prepared physician-executive, and (c) the task planner and the supervisor of the results, which are advantageous to have in a system.

We saw that human being has been preparing for artificial evolution, and over time, it will separate more and more from the environment it breeds and increasingly becomes the creator of its own ecological niche. The subject of evolutionary changes becomes the relationship with the environment; the means of evolution are 'superstructures' and 'improvements' of their bodies. It has become clear that these improvements will completely *change the lifestyles* and ways of socialisation of people in future.

We come to the conclusion about the future division of mankind on the basis of signs that led to the gradual formation of *two branches*:

> Long-living mankind with a high degree of readiness for the new, the desire for changes, and a 'milestone-modernised' body.

> Short-living mankind with a low degree of readiness for the new, fear of changes, and a sick, senile body.

Chapter 2

The Progress of Medical Technologies and Health Care Systems

I found a very interesting question about how the new medical technologies are changing the presentation of problems of HCS and vice versa, as well as how health care needs affect the development of medical technologies. In other words, how fast does the HCS detect the new tools in hands and begin to expand its tasks according these tools, and at the same time, how quickly HCS begins to invest in the development of new tools after it has a new challenge? I will begin this chapter with an attempt to understand why medical technology is different from all the others.

2. A. What's the Medical Technology?

Before recalling how medical technologies began, let's give the *definition of technology* in general:

> *Technology* (from the Greek téchne—art, skill, and Greek logos—study)—a set of methods and tools for achieving the desired result, the method of converting given into the necessary, the mode of production.

Technology was born when one inventor (no matter what he invented) recorded the thing he invented as a sequence of individual operations—exactly how to do it and how to get it right for everyone. That is, technology is the moment of transition from the individual art of one gifted man to mass production for the majority, which is endowed with a lot less by nature in this matter. The term *technology* was introduced in scientific use by Johann Bekkman (1739-1811), who described it as a scientific discipline at the German University of Goettingen in 1772.

Technologies in the methodology of the UN are divided into the following:

- *technology in its pure form, which covers methods and techniques of production of goods and services (dissembled technology);*
- *embodied technology, covering machinery, equipment, buildings, entire production systems, and products with high technical and economic parameters (embodied technology).*

Thus, it makes sense to divide the technology, including the medical one, into two types: technology as knowledge and technology as production capacity. Consider, just for simplicity of communication, that the first technology is named A, the second one is called B. The first technology (which is A) more often appears under the nickname of 'know-how' and it includes certain algorithms by which you can get the desired result, and as a rule, these algorithms do not follow directly from the knowledge known from the open literature but from the preliminary volume of research.

In general, the prepared reader uses technology A, but the prepared executive uses technology B. Technology B by definition may exist and work even without the presence of a developer. Roughly speaking, the prepared executive of technology B can produce a product that is none the worse than that made by the engineer-designer, i.e. knowledge of technology A is completely transferred into technology B, and in general the final result does not depend much on the user. In medicine, the situation is radically different: Medicine is still stubbornly called 'the art', and this is partly true, because it has long been observed that even in very advanced technology the low-trained user almost never can get the same result as the technologist-developer himself. The expected maximal result in medicine is obtained only if technology B organised by a customer is used, which at the training level it is a minimum equal to the developer of technology A. In terms of technological chain, it also means that medical technology A is usually never transferred completely into medical technology B and requires some additional virtual component, which we usually call 'clinical experience', 'school', 'medical intuition', and that can correctly interpret the result issued by technology B. At the household level, we call it 'art of medicine'. So the *first* feature of medical technology is as follows:

> To achieve the maximum result, the person who develops
> the medical technology and the end user should have an
> equal level of qualifications.

Further, unlike other technologies, medicine often cannot measure the achieved results. Figures in numerous tests and measurements of the organism often have no relationship to the real state of health of the customer-patient. Currently, we measure in medicine not what really should be measured, and that is technically measurable. To evaluate the achieved results, we need an interpreter-doctor who by indirect signs can assess the result, serving as a 'translator' between the patient and technology A, thus giving feedback, without which the progress of technology A is impossible. The problem is that the concept of success and failure of the application of technology B is very subjective and difficult to measure, which gives us a *second* feature of medical technology:

> Technology B in medicine always consists of two components: the actual production facilities and equipment on the one hand and non-formalised intellectual work to evaluate results on the other hand.

The third feature of medical technology is the subject of focus itself. Nowadays, we know ten times more of the structure and physiology of the human body than the great Lister knew and a thousand times more than that known by the great Galen. Mortality from most diseases and injuries was reduced in number, which physicians in the early twentieth century never dreamed of. But until now, medicine cannot ensure that medical manipulation or drug administration to one person gives exactly the same result as of any other person. Our bodies are different; they differ from each other with the not yet known details of physiology at the molecular level, and any attempt to organise a mindless conveyor production of medical services will still end more or less in a large percentage of failures. So far, all attempts to automate or to formalise the process of clinical decision failed. The *third* feature of medical technology is as follows:

The difference in the structure and physiology of the human body leads to the probabilistic nature of the results of application of medical technology B.

By the way, if you recall the development of technology in general, it is possible to draw analogies between the probabilistic nature of the results of medical technology B and the certain percentage of production rejects in manufacturing. Mankind faced the problem of production rejects at the beginning of the machinery period (starting from manufactories), when the performers could not follow the technology exactly because of the following:

- Poor quality of raw materials
- Inaccurate machines
- Failure to accurately calibrate the instruments
- Low-skilled executives.

As a solution to these problems, the quality control system was implemented, because of which the production reject is decreasing. Modern robotic production has reduced the reject rate to vanishingly small quantities. Ease in solving the problem of reject in production is largely due to the fact that the objects of production, tools, and measuring instruments—all of the objects—are produced by man. Structure and parameters of these objects are known in detail, at least at the level required for this production. In medicine, the reject rate with the application of technology B can be estimated as the sum of the following:

a) the characteristics of the person exposed—in other words, how much the patient's organism is *standard*;
b) *difficulties in calibration* as instruments of influence and instruments of result measurement;

c) the *difference in skills level* and discipline of executives (often the executive may be the patient himself who may be totally unprepared from a medical point of view);

d) variable and unpredictable *effects of environment* on the patient before, during, and after the treatment, distorting the achieved results;

e) *mutual influence* of several pathological processes in the human body, which are difficult to predict, some of which are not noticed by the physician or even by the patient;

There is one more feature of medical technology. What would you say about the part in the machine which has its own idea of what it should be? What should be the size and consumer properties? Is it easy to handle the part in the machine if each movement of the tool would be accompanied by the reaction of part itself? Namely in this way behaves the living organism while they try to apply the medical technology to it, i.e. the external technology superimposed on the body's own actions, aimed at both self-treatment of the pathological process and to counter external technological intervention, which the organism perceives as *injury*.

> The result of the application of medical technology B is a consequence of a proper external intervention, as well as the organism's reactions to the disease and to the intervention itself.

From this, it follows another obvious feature of medical technology: They are applied to continuously and rapidly changing live object, and the algorithm of these changes is extremely difficult and cannot be fully predicted at the current level of development of science. These changes depend on many factors:

- The age of the organism;
- The states of the nervous system as the control centre for this organism;
- Progress of the individual's biological clock, including jet lag;
- Powerful complex effects of unnatural chemicals that enter the body through food, beverages, cosmetics and toiletries, detergents, food additives, air, and unassigned medicines.
- Presence of abnormalities in the body that are not perceived by them as pathological but which alter the course of physiological processes. Of course, such deviations are not considered as pathological by medical technologists (even if they can find them, they are considered as 'variant of norm') and not recorded in history as diagnoses (because such nosological items do not exist yet) and therefore they do not affect the use of medical technology B to the given organism;
- Impact of natural factors, such as solar radiation, ambient temperature, Earth's magnetic field, the radiation surrounding the organism's appliances, inaudible ultrasounds issued by natural and artificial sources, variations in atmospheric pressure, natural and artificial radioactivity;
- Impact of other individuals of the same species, continuously in contact with the given organism because he is a social being and linked to all members of the community;
- Impact of individuals of other species, either permanently or temporarily residing within the organism, as well as on the surface of his body. They refer to viruses, protozoa, fungi, flat and round worms, tiny arthropods;
- Impact of other living beings, either permanently or temporarily residing with the human. They refer to the household and decorative animals affecting the human in contact with them and vice versa;
- Other exogenous and endogenous factors affecting the human body in ways yet unknown.

Thus, the following feature of medical technology is as follows:

> The target object of medical technology B is continuously and uncontrollably changing between the beginning and end of use of technology.

Finally, the last feature of medical technology: It is fully described by a special section of law—medical legislation. Imagine a group of parts which together make up the rules for handling themselves: how and on which machines, how long, and how many resources it is permissible to spend. It's clear that all of the medical technology will be a reflection of the moral imperatives of the community of these parts, and no one technology that falls out from it can develop in such a community. Thus:

> Range of possible solutions for the development and application of medical technologies is under strict legal control of the target objects of these technologies.

In summary, *characteristics* of medical technology in simple terms can be described as follows:

- Medical technology cannot be applied correctly by simply doing the listed actions. You must understand what it is doing and why. And you also need to know what to do if things were to go 'very wrong', as a health care worker cannot just discard spoiled detail. He is forced to finish the process for each object.
- The results of medical technology can be properly assessed only by a trained specialist, but not by a client, who is the target object of the application of this technology.
- One should understand the probabilistic nature of the result.

- The reaction of the living target object on the use of medical technology B is an integral part of the total result of its application.
- Medical technology B, in contrast to other manufacturing technologies, is applied to the dynamic target object, and this object changes in unpredictable ways during the production cycle.
- The area of possible technological solutions in medicine is artificially narrowed according to the current moral imperatives of society, whose negative points affect the speed of development of such technology.

If we consider the medical technologies in terms of the completeness of solving a problem, it becomes apparent that their character is changing over time. In the early development of medicine, the treatment technologies did not solve problems at all (instead, they changed attitude to customer problems) or eliminated only some of the symptoms of the problem. Real effective methods of the treatment of certain diseases can be counted on fingers. From the point of view of today's science, none of the ancient methods can be considered effective. Mankind used them when the cause of the problem could not be understood on the basis of scientific knowledge; namely, the decision could not be effective. So as to not sit on one's hands, people simulated the solution of the problem; especially given the fact that in the medical sense the problem sometimes got really solved itself, through self-healing. I suggest that such technologies should be called *imitations*.

With the accumulation of scientific facts and improving the methodology for obtaining them, medical technologies also have changed; they are no longer engaged in the struggle of separating symptoms, but they try to solve the problem entirely. The difficulty was that there was no unified theory of processes in the human body and understanding that the issue at hand (disease) is a manifestation of more general processes. But at the level of individual organs, for a time such treatment technologies worked. I suggest naming such medical technology as intermediate, since their results are really *intermediate*; it acts for one organ and/or only for a while. On closer examination, most of today's medical technologies are intermediate because they require constant repetition of therapeutic actions and/or close monitoring by specialists for applying this technology to prevent recurrence or complications of the disease.

But today we can see that medical technologies that *solve the problem at its root* are starting to emerge. Their distinguishable features are as follows:

- *Wide application*: Medical problems are solved completely in the majority of subjects of this species.
- *Spot effects*: They affect only those systems or body organs that require medical intervention. That is, the side effects of technology are even absent (below the current threshold of measurement) or they can be ignored, since they are fully compensated by the body.
- *Final effect*: They do not require repetition of medical procedures and provide lifelong results for a given organism.
- *Versatility*: Often they do not operate on only one issue, but on a whole class of similar problems (a group of nosological items).
- *Irreversibility*: The reversion of the organism is not possible; that is, the result of the application of such technology cannot be undone.

One of the first such technologies, found almost by accident, was the smallpox vaccination (Edward Jenner, 1796). After this procedure, the person will never in his life been sick with smallpox, but undoing the vaccination was impossible. I suggest naming such a medical technology as *closing* or *final*. When an organism uses it, the organism is changing forever in such a way that that particular disease does not occur or the external causative agent cannot damage the body.

The only disadvantage of *closing* technology is that the result is not inherited. As soon as we find a way to consolidate the achieved results also for the descendants of the given person, i.e. make meaningful and controllable changes in the genome of this species, the technology will be *perfect*; that is, it eliminates the problem forever.

In the next chapter, we will talk about why mankind is currently experiencing a feeling that medicine has always fallen short of its needs. All the time, there is a lack of quantity and quality of medical services; all the time, there is some conflict between the public and health professionals and this is not observed in other technological fields and industries.

2. B. Medical Technology As a Religious Procedure

What exactly do I mean by that?

If we recall how scientific knowledge began, the first thing that we find in textbooks is that each branch of knowledge once grew out of the contradictions between the religious views of the world and accumulated the real facts. Out of the contradictions between the world picture offered by the Catholic Church and the facts that people saw in the sky, modern European astronomy was born, having the first child period under the title 'astrology'. At the same time, similar contradictions were born: chemistry (alchemy) and physics (natural philosophy). When naturalists modestly collecting plants, lizards, beetles, and birds' eggs in a remote corner of the world saw that species were continually changing, modern biology was born. The usual treasure hunters, who found discrepancies between the Old Testament and the pictures they saw in the excavation, turned into modern archaeologists, etc. How was medicine born? I propose we start from the beginning.

Ability of self-healing and self-treating is one of the most ancient mechanisms of living beings. When all life on Earth consisted of a 'soup' presented in the form of organic molecules floating in proto-ocean, the initial sign of living consisted of the ability to copy 'oneself beloved' out of scrap materials as many times as possible. The habitats of these molecules have been extremely favourable environments for them from the chemical point of view. With increasing number of beings wanting to be copied, the amount of anybody's construction material in the area decreased, so competing began for (a) building materials and (b) habitat. As soon as the competition appeared, ways of taking away the resources from each other materialised and it so hard that both fighting parties incurred serious injuries. Attempts to go beyond the usual habitat also caused the damages of the structure (can easily imagine your own number of damaging factors). At this point, the ability to recover from injury or illness becomes a sign of living; it becomes a key requirement of procreation and expansion into other habitats. The opportunity to repair itself has allowed life on Earth to dramatically increase the average lifespan of all species, enabling them to learn more about the environment and produce more conditioned reflexes for the survival of each species and to shape them into instincts over time and pass them on to their progeny in the ready-to-use form.

With the complexity of the structure of the body and improvement in the functions of its organs and tissues, there was the standard reaction to self-treatment. It makes sense that such reactions are divided into intracellular (molecular level), intercellular (tissue level), and the organism as a whole (organs' level). To coordinate these reactions, the nervous system developed the whole chains of signals, conjugating these responses into something meaningful, and that achieved the goals. As the highest level of coordination the behavioural response that was specific to each species emerged, and that increased the chances of survival of any particular individual or group of individuals in general (for herd animals). Well, as the pinnacle of behavioural responses to illness and injuries among our distant ancestors, they made an effort to help their own body (and their neighbour's body) to recover. According to A. P. Nazaretyan, the investigation at the intersection point of archaeology, ethnography, cultural anthropology, psychology, and neurophysiology (Davidenkov, 1947; Pfeiffer, 1982; Rozin, 1999; Grimak, 2001), showed that 'the direction of selection miraculously changed: happens an expansion of hysteroid psychasthenic persons with increased liability, suggestibility, unnaturally developed imagination and a tendency to neurotic fears. In a few herds, where the individuals of this type were dominated, the first artificial (above instinct) mechanisms of inhibition of intraspecific aggression were formed. Such a mechanism was the necrophobia—pathological fear of the corpses, which were attributed to the ability to arbitrary actions. Neurotic fear of posthumous revenge is not only limited the murder within the herd, but also stimulated the biologically non-distinctive concern for the maimed and non-viable relatives and ritual behaviour with the dead body'. Good solutions for self- and mutual treatment were accidently found secured in the form of tradition. No one knew why these decisions were successful; because of the lack of any scientific methodology, the tradition turned into a question of faith and merged with religious rites, which emerged later.

Religious medical procedure passed down from generation to generation as a tradition had a progressive meaning because in those times, when writing was not there, the only way to save information was by word of mouth; it was more so important that one obtained with blood and death of their fellow tribesmen, to 'hang' this information with religious meaning and 'sanctify' it with that. Thus, the medical knowledge 'working' part of which consisted mainly of herbs, taking certain substances of mineral and biological origin found in nature and protective regime; it went forward to the ancient times where they began to be recorded, but were still not separated from the issue of faith. A period of temple medicine started. Primitive surgical skills were the sole responsibility of barbers; they considered it a dirty job and it had nothing to do with religion, I think, because there was a clear and obvious link between the action and the results achieved. The divinity was just nowhere to be put. In this form, medicine survived until the late Middle Ages.

Renaissance was characterised also by, among other events, separation of religious and scientific world, although all the scholars of that time were deeply religious people. The facts do not fit into the religious worldview flooding the world, causing resistance from the church. But as soon as science began to give practical results, i.e. from a simple 'philosophising' it started to gain industrial strength—the resistance of the church authorities gradually disappeared. The development of medicine in this time dramatically slowed compared to other sciences because of so were many reasons:

- Centuries' old religious ban on the study of anatomy of the human body on corpses delayed development of medical thought in Europe for long. European and Arab doctors studied anatomy through the works of Galen done centuries ago.
- Development of biology in general, in particular medicine, was strongly inhibited because of the lack of scientific tools for studying biological objects. In fact, medicine during all this time remained an ancient narrative discipline, like history and geography. Experiment in medicine was largely absent.
- Physics and chemistry used the mathematical techniques in full, which were already very well developed, but in medicine it cannot be applied because of the inability to measure and express in figures the parameters of the human body.
- There was no general theory of the human body processes.

This weakness of medicine was felt greatly by contemporaries. In Europe, jokes and cartoons crept in about stupid and greedy doctors who wrinkled their foreheads on imaginary problems instead of the real ones. It was a general impression that the physicians, in contrast to real scientists, did nonsense. And this was largely true—medicine in that time was still a set of religious procedures hallowed with tradition and was not a science at all.

Grandiose breaking of public consciousness occurred only after the recognition of Darwin's theory in the mid-nineteenth century, when mankind realised with great difficulty that the human body was constructed and operated on the same principles as the bodies of all animals. It is difficult to imagine the indignation and surprise that people felt at that time when they realise themselves that they were 'rational animal'. Almost immediately after these events, the gradual separation of biomedical facts from the religious understanding that man was God's creation began.

And just at that moment began the emergence of professional scientists in the modern sense of the word 'scientist', who worked in the medical field where up till now the criterion of truth was the religious dogma and tradition, as a form of such dogma. At the end of the nineteenth century, the criterion of truth in medicine became a practice, which serviced the interests of a completely new social phenomenon—the *clinic*.

As is well known from school textbooks, the first institutions for treatment and care of the sick and wounded in Europe were the inns, created by the military religious orders (especially hospitallers) in the path of pilgrims going to the Holy Land and back. At the end of the eleventh century, they organised a network of hospitals and asylums in many countries of Europe and the Holy Land—in Antioch, Jerusalem, and other cities of the East. One of the first was John the Merciful hospital in Jerusalem at the beginning of the twelfth century, which was able to accept up to 2,000 patients and even had a special department for the treatment of eye diseases. This was the first place where Europeans could see patients in mass, follow the mass patients' response to the same treatment actions and view statistics. They were, so to speak, medical manufactories, i.e. places of mass production of medical services, which were exclusively produced individually before. We must also say that they were free institutions; their clients came from all segments of society then, as all Christians, regardless of their social status, felt it necessary to at least once in their life make a pilgrimage, as those who saw the picture of illness and recovery in such institutions had rather a representative sample, which were equally represented in all ages and states of society. It's important for us to note that these hospitals-manufactories (unlike all the other manufactories, such as wool) were religious institutions existing on the money of monastic orders, were often beyond the walls of monasteries with strict statute, and acted exactly in the mainstream of contemporary Roman Catholic dogma.

Manufactories that produced goods for the market existed in the market conditions and readily used all achievements of contemporary science and invention to obtain greater profits. Medical manufactories-hospitals were deprived of this, as their products did not come out in the market, as well as medical science, even in its infancy, was not allowed in religious institutions and monasteries. It is not surprising that in a few hundred years a significant lag in results in practical applications of biomedical knowledge from the results of the technical one had accumulated. Catholic Europe was far behind in medicine than the non-Christian world, particularly the East, where religion from the outset would not interfere in the development of science. If you recall the medieval European fairy tales, you will observe with surprise that such a character like a doctor usually appeared in a turban and robe. And it was true: Almost all of European doctors in the early Dark Ages were represented by wandering and court Arab scholars (mostly from Muslim countries of Maghreb and Iberian Peninsula). The dominance of Arab scientists was so much that even the translations of works of Galen were distributed in Arabic. The next generation of European physicians (somewhere in the fourteenth to fifteenth century) were already Christians, but the conditions were so that doctors existed separately from hospitals, just like the religious institutions behind the monastery walls. This lag in medicine persisted until the early nineteenth century.

During major wars of the nineteenth century that captured areas of whole continents and resulted in unprecedented losses, including a crowd of wounded and sick people with long treatment periods, led to the fact that religious institutions set up for the care and treatment of those suffering ceased to cope with the flow of customers, both physically and financially. States really began to feel the demographic and social consequences of their military exercises. Saving the population of their countries had become imperative for all the warring states, which led to drastic changes in the attitude of the state to hospitals and military medicine in general. Monastic medicine spilled beyond the walls of monasteries; a new social phenomenon appeared—nurses; with this, their religious component gradually went out and medical professionalism remained.

Thus, military hospitals formed, despite the fact that they were mostly mobile and demanded that the conveyer provide similar medical services. This started the specialisation of doctors and their assistants. The sharply increased demands for quality treatment, because the simple care and enhanced food were not enough for the effective execution of the tasks assigned by the state. All the decisions, which had shown its effectiveness, were implemented; the new methods of treatment were tested immediately; the wounded soldiers were 'rabbits', on which the military surgeons were improving their skills. The more the military medicine fought for efficiency (and achieved it!), the less the religious traditions and ceremonies remained in medicine. The last remaining religious procedure that was possible to be seen in the modern hospital was the rite performed over the dying hopeless patient, and that too at his request.

Thus, we can say that medicine as a practical production of health care services has only relatively recently emerged from under the guardianship of the religious consciousness and traditions and swiftly made up for the time it was accumulated over several centuries behind the other fundamental disciplines. Laws that describe the limitations and scope of the activities of physicians and biologists (as opposed to other sciences) are the reflection of religious public morality of past centuries and are constantly in conflict with society's needs and capabilities of medical science. The resolving of this controversy, I think, would dramatically accelerate the progress of medical science and would give mankind the opportunities which it has long dreamed of.

In the next section, we will talk about carriers of medical technologies and how they pass their knowledge to each other.

2. C. Does the Medical Technology Exist Without Doctors?

The question is akin to this: Can there be aviation industry if you do not have any pilot? The answer would seem clear. Indeed, if we have already described that for correct application of medical technology it is necessary for developer-technologist and executive to have an equal training level, what can still be the issue? Questions really are the following:

- How to define the medical technology and distinguish it from any other? And why do we need to know we deal with medical technology?
- How to consider the use of medical technology by unqualified executives?
- How to identify a suitably qualified executive of a particular technology, in particular, if the developer is out of touch?
- And, in general, whom do we mean when we say 'without doctors'?
- What should we do if it's impossible to find a skilled executive of given technology at all?

So let's define the concept of *medical technology*. From the previous chapter, it became clear that there are numerous differences between medical technologies and others, but for a definition, we need to select the main signs. I propose the following definition:

> *Medical technology* is a combination of knowledge, skills, techniques, and equipment that enable a qualified specialist to affect the natural development and changes of biological objects directly or indirectly, both individually and en masse, taking into account the

reaction of the objects themselves and achieving goals with the greatest degree of probability. At a certain point, it becomes a tool for the *health care system*.

This definition describes all of the above most significant signs of medical technology, and just like the above definition of medicine, it is not tied to the notion of 'human'. Then what are the distinguishing factors between 'medicine' and 'medical technology'? Both definitions speak of knowledge and skills. I think the difference is that 'technology' is written (in the form of specific procedures and equipment) knowledge, i.e. knowledge that can be used to achieve goals right now. 'Medicine' is a much broader concept; it includes both medical technologies and the knowledge that can be used for other purposes if they would change or be subject to refinement, i.e. knowledge that can be transferred into technologies in certain conditions. Also, 'medicine' includes the training of specialists, using and developing medical technologies, i.e. technology of development technologies. We can also say that medical technology is a 'cast of medicine', meaning that it is ready to be used for solving problems at the moment. If problem changes, another 'cast' will be made. As we discovered earlier, tasks will be delivered by a more general structure—the health care system (HCS).

Understanding the nature of medical technologies, their features, and limitations, it's seems to me necessary to the following:

- Proper application of the available medical technologies.
- Tracking the time when the changed tasks require changing the technologies.
- Maintenance of the structures that develop new medical technologies for new challenges, including the 'rainy days'.
- Correct expectations from the use of given technologies and monitoring its outcomes.

- Limiting the range of professionals who have the right to use medical technologies.
- Public control over the professionals that apply them.
- Public control over the appearance and use of medical technologies that do not fit (or do not fit more) in the tasks set by the HCS.

Proceeding forward from the fact that medical technologies require training for its correct application and understanding of the results of this application, the HCS as a state superstructure is trying to limit the number of people who are allowed to use them, otherwise no monitoring is possible.

History of the state's understanding that the medical technologies and their application are vital to control is old enough. Initially, as we recall, the state did not interfere in the physician-patient relationship. In those days, everyone who wanted to do it and passed an individual course of study with a more or less well-known colleague were called doctors. We can say that man became a doctor by recognition of the community, i.e. those who had seen firsthand the results of his work. Due to lack of scientific methodology and criteria, it was impossible to distinguish the charlatan from the real doctor, and an entirely illiterate population (including the elite) judged the activities of doctors only on the principle of 'I do believe him, but this one—no'.

The situation changed after universities appeared in the medieval Europe, which started to issue diplomas to its graduates. For some time, there weren't special medical diplomas (as well as in other specialties); diplomas were universal, i.e. universities produced experts with 'very broad' profiles. They began to apply the word 'doctor' (Latin *doctor*—teacher, mentor, from 'docere' (Lat. 'to teach')), meaning a learned man, as opposed to simply 'medico' or 'chiropractor'. Attributes that confirm the qualifications are quite funny in today's time:

22 May 1537: Francois Rabelais received the highest academic title of doctor of medicine in University of Montpellier (with the award of a gold ring, embossed gold sash, panama hats from the black drapes, hats of crimson silk and copied the works of Hippocrates). And the state of Rabelais, before highly questionable (he was a runaway monk and a few years was in hiding), has become one of the most enviable and listed attributes of the doctor from afar, all pointing to the special privileges of their owner.

Generally, it can be said that the medieval university culture evolved not only as non-governmental but also to some extent as anti-government opposition, the super-national culture level. If you recall the administrative and legal autonomy of universities, the common language of teaching and publication of scientific works—Latin, the free pan-European labour market for professors, and the common market of knowledge for students—then the idea of the Bologna system of education comes up. Doctors who were issued in such a way were ready to practice in any city of any European country; *they no longer had to spend time and efforts to prove their expertise in the given community.* At the same time, potential patients were fast and reliable way to distinguish a true expert of charlatan. That is, in fact, medicine became the first internationally licensed profession, to enter the market of which required not only talent, knowledge, and skills but also a formal proof of qualification issued by an authoritative institution. It is important to say that universities had no connection to states (despite the fact that some of them were founded by the monarchs and their contributions) and that the diplomas and titles were assigned not on behalf of the state or monarch, but namely on behalf of the scientific community the university (faculty). Just as the medieval master put the stamp on his product of an approved sample by guild, confirming the time and place of manufacture and authorship, universities as well 'branded' their products with diplomas, preventing the penetration of 'fakes' in the market.

When Europe entered the industrial era, all the states needed professionals of such quality and in such quantities that old self-governing universities failed to provide. States began to establish their own new universities, and their diplomas already had state status. In the labour market, both varieties of diplomas were on equal terms. At some stage, the state realised that technology was a strategic thing, especially the medical technologies that give an advantage to the most important: the quality and quantity of the population. And the states found a way to control the use of medical technologies: They created the legislative field, aimed solely at doctors and their relationships with patients. No other profession has won much attention of the state in terms of restrictions and control over their activities as medicine (including sanitation), and it is not surprising—because *the entire population passes through the hands of health care workers.* Tight control over qualification and the number of doctors was usually performed by state licensing after the implementation of certain conditions—the qualifying examination. Thus, the use of medical technologies by the 'not allowed' person becomes an obvious offense that is easy suppressible. Interests of patients who clearly needed additional quantity of doctors have been ignored by the state since it was believed that the issues of controlling the spread of medical technologies were far more important than vital needs of individual patients.

Division of medicine into conventional and traditional categories did not change anything, in fact, because the government immediately imposed separate licenses for both. If another type of medicine will appear, the government once again will come up with a way to restrict it and put in the legal framework. States unequivocally believe that the use of medical technologies by people they (the states) cannot control is dangerous to themselves. I think that these subconscious fears grow when medical technologies become more powerful and their obvious consequences are seen more and more, but at the same time, their long-term consequences are difficult to predict. Quite logically, all states continuously enhance the level of control over the quantity and quality of doctors, and it is already noticeable that the more technologically developed country, the more strongly it tends to control the use of medical technologies in its territory. But a metre away from the state boundary they are powerless, so the patient can always find the 'lax controlled' doctor for medical services that he still wants to get. There's the inevitable moment when the states will be forced to collude to control the medical technologies because there is no sense in controlling them within state borders if the object of their application—people—move freely between countries in the globalised world.

How do the states determine the qualifications of physicians implementing technology B are sufficient? The qualifying examination involves the comparison of knowledge and skills of the applicant with a certain standard. The standard is the collective developer of technology A, which annually accounts for a new version of the exam and methodically and consistently adjusts the qualifications of physicians under his current understanding of the issue, filtering out those who understand it's not like he did. Note that it is not 'better' or 'worse', but, namely, 'not like he did'. Such a system is more or less valid if the medical qualifying examination is regularly compiled by the 'collective technology A developer', and the results of medical technology on average will be no worse (but also will not improve until another technology with another 'examiner' will be offered). The results of the technology use 'freeze' on the same level and wait for the other medical technology that is more efficient in terms of its nature. A much more sad result can be seen when the qualifying exam takes someone who understands technology A 'in a wrong way', unlike a true developer. In general, this situation occurs during the following:

- the real developer is too expensive for the given state,
- the technology itself is too expensive or requires specialised knowledge and processes (equipment) beyond the current capabilities of the given state,
- the developer is represented by a single man who physically cannot be 'examiner' for the entire mass of applicants,
- the developer refuses to publish full details of his developed technology for any reason,
- The developer dies without leaving an exhaustive guide.

In circumstances when the standard is incorrect, an inevitably massive and steady decline of qualifications of medical personnel occurs, resulting in the deterioration of the use of technology B which becomes unacceptable for a given state; after that the technology is limited to being used within the state and is recognised as 'ineligible' by the local medical community. Such 'misunderstood' medical technology becomes, therefore, a time bomb for a given state, and then we have the inevitable moment when new technology based on this one appears, which is more efficient but less clear, and attempts to use that which would be so much ineligible by local unskilled personnel that it would be refused by the highest level of management.

Therefore, with each innovation the technological backwardness of the given state *increases*. Renunciation of the use of more efficient medical technologies and misunderstanding their benefits inevitably sooner or later leads to a *lag in quality and quantity of the population*. The situation is complicated by the fact that nowadays the number of innovations is steadily increasing and the timing of technology change is shortened all the time so that states have fallen behind (for whatever reason), deprived of the opportunity to catch up with process in a natural way. A situation arises when the import of technologies and equipment in the given country becomes useless, because there are no such experts, which the given state would recognise as qualified, so new technologies should be brought together with the skilled personnel, the qualifications of which the given state can no longer control. If this happens, this state will lose control over the use of medical technologies in its territory; that is, the whole system of training and licensing of in-house medical specialists would have no longer practical sense and would turn to tradition, some conventional rite. Such a state would be forced to accept someone else's system of certification of medical specialists.

To answer the question posed in the beginning of the chapter 'Can medical technology exist without doctors?', in the present level of development it should be 'yes, but this technology cannot be applied'; therefore, its existence does not make any economic sense. By analogy with the dead languages, for which we know not a single living carrier, it makes sense to introduce the concept of *dead medical technology*. 'Dead' can be called a technology that you know exists, but the carrier of it does not exist or is not available in the given environment. *Dead medical technology* can be described in detail, even may have full technical support and documentation, but in the absence of a qualified carrier it becomes just a historical socio-cultural artefact, by analogy with the Latin or Greek languages, which are *dead* despite the availability of detailed vocabularies and abundance of people who know how to read these dictionaries.

Thus, the simple arguments about the nature of the medical technologies have led us to an understanding of how the states for any reasons hopelessly lagging behind in medical technologies and training for medical personnel in today's globalised world face a tragic choice: Either they are completely closed for the world and watch the slow decline of its population or allow developers of more effective medical technologies to *control the quality and quantity of people* on its territory.

2. D. What's the Product of Medical Technologies?

Indeed, all the technologies produce something, either products or services. As we explained in the previous chapter, any medical technology makes *purposeful changes in the state of biological objects*. Calling this 'product' is difficult; apparently, it's the 'service' nevertheless. Goods being produced somehow have the ability to circulate between consumers and change their value. Medical service does not have this property: It cannot be arbitrarily transferred from one consumer to another; it is always targeted. It can be argued that the medicines, medical equipment, etc. are products which are necessary for the application of medical technology. But all these things are the embodied technology B required to produce the above changes. That is, the final product is the service again. But service to whom? And who pays for it? And if you pay, then what?

It is logical to assume that the customer of 'targeted changes in biological objects' is the one to whom these changes are beneficial, and the notion of benefit for modern technology can stretch into the future for a long time, which may exceed the lifetime of the current generation. It is clear that when a patient (agreed that we are talking about the working man) comes to the medical establishment, he admits that he wishes to alter the condition of the body (or the body of his child) because of the following:

- He cannot work/study because of disease.
- The disease/injury threatens his life.
- He wants to improve their quality of life.
- He wants to improve his body (for any reason).

Thus, we can say that the production of medical technology is *changing the individual patient's body to preserve his life, eliminating pathological focus to the point of being comfortable, allowing him to work as well as showing some improvement in his body*. It is important to say that for solving these problems a certain range of medical technologies that have been developed in advance can be applied. These days nobody will develop a special medical technology for the specific (even vital) needs of a single patient or a small group of patients. Patient-customer pays for service he needs (in this case it does not matter which way) from that range of services that are ready (allowed) to be used at the moment and have the necessary consumer properties.

A completely different relationship occurs when the entire mass of potential patients form a public inquiry and through a representative (state agency) express a desire to apply a medical technology to himself aimed at

- facilitating the flow (or full prevention) of already known illnesses/injuries,
- preventing new (or re-emerging) diseases,
- improving their bodies to get certain benefits.

It is logical to assume that this is the case of *mass* changing of organisms, but interest in this case is not individual; some persons even may be against it, but there is group interest, namely, to obtain certain advantages compared with other groups. It is important to understand that this technology cannot exist beforehand (because there was no demand for it); it will have to develop specifically for this task and it will have to pay for the entire group as a whole, taking into account the risk of failure. The final product of this technology is *an advantage over other individuals competing for a given economic or ecological niche*.

It becomes clear here that in the first case beneficiary of the use of technology becomes a patient-customer individually paying for a standard medical service. In the second case, the beneficiary is a large group of potential patients; ideally, the entire population of the state collectively pays for the development and application of new technology to produce some benefits for the entire group.

In both cases, products of medical technology lead to changes in living organisms, but their purpose is different: In the first case, it is to change the single organism to obtain individual competitive advantages; in the second one it is to change all individuals of a given population to gain a competitive advantage at the level of species.

Payment for use of technology also differs: In the *first* case, the money for the use of ready-made technology by a particular patient—the amount known in advance due to market demand and supply—passes from the patient or the money accumulator (health insurance company or other) to the owner of the medical technology (doctor, medical institution), who is trying to commercially justify his efforts to develop (acquisition) of the technology. So we have an act of sale (albeit in instalments) between a customer and a seller.

In the *second* case, for the development of medical technology necessary for the public, unknown they spend an advance amount of those funds that do not belong to the citizens and are paid in various forms to the state (as the superstructure of society) in taxes by the current generation of patients and all earlier patients. Also, it includes funds that the state has earned itself on behalf of the population, but is forced to spend them at the request of the society. That is, in this case no sales happens, because patients cannot buy technologies that belong to themselves. And once the sale does not occur, then the market concept in this case is irrelevant.

What does the beneficiary pay in each case? In the first case, he pays the money (remember, we are talking about a working member of society) accumulated by him personally, his parents, and close relatives, gaining for them a better and longer life. In the second case, the beneficiary invests part of the social product, which had already existed in monetary and non-monetary forms, to promote the quality of the population and, ultimately, to increase the production of this social product.

In the next section, we will review the main benefits of the presence of modern HCS to the public.

2. E. Is It Possible to Live without Health Care System?

That's a strange question. And how did society live before the formalised health care system, such as the advanced society of Roman Empire in the first century BC or the Meiji restoration in Japan? Moreover, the population in these times was even growing, so these periods in the life of different countries were examples of flourishing culture and even the Golden Age . . . Why did the society not feel the lack of the health care system (even if they knew such a thing) as a drawback, yet now the country without a health care system is perceived as defective, as a failed state?

As mentioned above, the health system appears at a certain stage of development of society, when it recognises the need for stimulation to increase the quantity and quality of the population. What is meant by quality of the population? This is an entirely separate question; more important is that the current state of the population did not satisfy the society, and it agreed to *invest the part of the social product in people*, hoping to get from this some strategic advantage. What makes the state, at some stage, take care about the quality of its population?

- I think that it is the *presence of a strong neighbour-competitor*, which leads one to think about the social system to improve the quality and quantity of the population. And the competition can take place as a purely military contest, so can the technological and even the demographic one.
- It has a significant value the *way of social production*, i.e. by which the growth of resource happens. If the main production and labour resource is the worker-slave, who can capture the battle in the neighbouring territory (Asian or slave mode of production), it is no use to take care of the slaves there, until there is an influx from outside. Slaves at this level of manual technology are interchangeable, so there is no need to worry about their quality. As the main

resource for growth is the machine (*mechanical slave*), which has a concept of efficiency in comparison with a competitor, for the first time there is a need for qualified technology providers and workers-executives. But the number of people is still an important parameter because neighbours, who are equal to the economic potential, taking advantage of the large number, are threatened by absorption.

- The emergence of nation states with clear borders and the institution of citizenship has led to the securing of the population within the territories; in the short historical period, it made sense in the *stimulation of the population* to protect their lands, but only as long as the amount of natural resources is allowed to feed the growing population. At this stage, the national health systems start to develop as a means to increasing the population of the country by reducing mortality.

- With the complexity of technology, the *number of employed workers ceases to have meaning* (it may even decrease), but sharply increases the demand for quality of workers. The quality of the population, its 'technological advancement', becomes more important parameter than its quantity.

- Further progress of technology leads to the fact that there is no need for large areas and natural resources on them; they can be either produced synthetically or purchased from a neighbour in a civilised way. There is a disappearing sense of territorial conquest and maintenance of large armies. The *number of people to maintain the army is no longer a strategic asset*, but the importance of its quality is further enhanced. Stimulation fertility recedes into the background before being prepared to attract specialists needed for economic growth from abroad.

- Further, national states are beginning to abandon the national principle so that the nation's flow is free between the countries; the population is globalising, leading to the fact that the state does not attract the population by its military power and size, but by the social standards and cleanliness of the territory. It is at this stage that the HCS of various countries is moving to a new quality: The results of their work are valuable not only in themselves, but also as a *competitive advantage in attracting people to the country*, not any, but that which is corresponding to the certain requirements. Without prior arrangement, the interstate selection of population begins, which leads to the fact that in some countries a more healthy and 'technologically advanced' population accumulates and gives offspring, giving a sharp economic growth; in contrast to them, in other countries it remains a painfully 'technologically backward' population.

- With the *competitive advantages* that attract the 'quality' population to the country are on one side and those that not allow him to leave the country on the other side, health systems can offer the following:

  - Advances in the treatment of the most common diseases that give the highest percentage mortality
  - Quality, ubiquity, and accessibility of emergency
  - Quality of paediatric care
  - Quality of care mothers and low infant mortality
  - The quality of health and social care to the elderly
  - The victory over infectious diseases at the level at which they do not turn into an epidemic (collective immunity of the population)
  - Availability of all of these types of care at a cost to the majority of population.

The modern interstate competition for a healthy and high-quality population, perceived by them as the main factor of scientific and technological progress, takes place in various forms and with varying intensity, depending on how strong is the difference between the rival states; as far as mobility of populations is concerned, what are the features of immigration policy and legislation, the degree of cultural unity and much more? But it is difficult to deny the fact that many states are already 'filtered' migrants by some known medical parameters. *States with the advanced medicine and health care system, of course, want the population to come to them to be treated, but have no interest in all the morbid people who will gather from around the globe for a permanent residence in their territory.*

States with similar approaches to the problem and with a similar control system form a community that in fact make their populations 'common' and allow him to freely 'flow' between these countries, including the treatment purposes. So does the European Union, and so do the United States and Canada. There is some kind of *medical cooperation* between such countries, while the shared population may choose the health care system of the country, which it currently enjoys and finds it more comfortable; there are areas of medical science in which the treatment of specific diseases is of better quality and at a lower cost abroad, while the home country does not make a tragedy of this, knowing that it compensates for the shortage in something that can do better.

Replying to a question posed in the title: 'Can you live without health care system?' it should be immediately clarified 'when?' and 'how long?'. If we are talking about the present time, the situation looks like this: A country with unformed health system and inadequate medicine will become the *donor of healthy populations* for countries with advanced health care systems. Within these undeveloped countries, the percentage of patient (unhealthy) population increases, firstly, because a healthy population gets sick and does not receive adequate care, and secondly, because a healthy population travels to countries where there is a chance to live longer, and an unhealthy person cannot do so as the developed country restricts their immigration in the medical sense. Quality of the population in a country rapidly deteriorates, economic growth stops, and the business becomes impossible due to lack of manpower and sufficient number of buyers; the territory of the state becomes almost empty, after which the state de facto *ceases to exist*, becoming a formality at the level of representation in international organisations.

The next section will raise the question: What is the difference between health care systems and what we call 'types of health care systems'?

2. F. Types of Health Care Systems, Do They Exist?

The first among the national health systems was the German model, created by Chancellor Otto von Bismarck in 1881. It served for improving the health of workers, who were seen as potential soldiers. The social insurance funds were initially created to pay for expenses for treatment and to give unemployment benefits, pensions, etc.; gradually the health insurance spun off. They received two-thirds of the sum at their disposal from employees and one-third from employers. Further, these institutions merged to form insurance companies, and the structure of employer contributions became dominant. Such a model still serves as a basis for public health in Germany and some other countries.

The form of payment for the service was changed as well. Rooted in the beginning since royalty, this principle was replaced with a more progressive method of payment for services in scores. While the first method stimulated the appointment of unnecessary, costly procedures, the second allowed you to adjust spending on health by paying the amount to doctors for the number of points earned, based on the results of treatment.

The system of Beveridge started in England in 1911 and was quickly endorsed by almost a third of the population. The system introduced by Prime Minister David Lloyd George had a distinctive feature that has survived to the present. Payment to physicians depended on the number of registered patients he served. The basic principle of payment of 'money follows the patient' leaving them with the free choice of doctor and the amount of the fee depended on the number of patients, gender, age, and social status. For the elderly, children under four years, women of childbearing age, and residents of poor neighbourhoods, payments were higher. Capitation payment also included facilities for inpatient treatment that prevented unwarranted hospitalisation in cases where home treatment was more effective and cheaper. It was believed that such a system encouraged a general practitioner to carry out preventive work, as it was cheaper than fighting the effects of the disease that had already developed.

In 1948, the labour government approved the reconstructed Beveridge system based on universal free health care. The calculation of Beveridge that free public medicine will treat patients better and lead to lower health care costs was utopian. The costs, however, increased by several times. Requirements of health care for patients increased dramatically as soon as it became apparent that they would not have to pay for treatment. Doctors began to shape the demand and supply in a completely unregulated environment: Often people with healthy teeth, twenty sealed teeth can be found, glasses are prescribed to people with normal vision, and appendectomy was performed totally for preventive purposes.

In Russia in 1912, a system of social insurance by Bismarck was introduced; it provided material support for workers during illness and for disabilities as a result of accidents. About 20% of workers were insured in the country. In general, the state preferred public health measures and improved sanitation and control of infectious diseases, which were not actually medical care. The number of medical facilities, doctors, and nurses was insufficient to meet the needs of the population. Thus, in 1913, for 6,900 residents of the Russian Empire there was one doctor, per 1,000 people there were 1.3 hospital beds, and medical institutions were distributed extremely unevenly in the country.[1]

During the First World War and the Civil War, the subsequent famine and mass epidemic gave public health and health care a crushing blow: Many medical facilities were physically destroyed, human losses were enormous, and the burden on health care increased for a long time. Shortly after the October Revolution,

---

[1]   Tragakes, E. and Lessof, S. In: Tragakes E., ed. *Health Care Systems in Transition*, Russian Federation: Copenhagen, *European Observatory on Health Care Systems*, 2003: 5(2).

only typhus (the epidemic that swept away 20-30 million people) killed three million people. N. Semashko participated in creating the recovery programme of health care and the foundation of the Soviet health system was laid, which declared his principles:

- Full responsibility of the state of health
- Accessibility of free health care
- Prevention of social diseases
- State control over the quality of medical care
- Close coordination of medical science and practice
- Unity in health promotion, treatment, and rehabilitation.

Based on these principles, the state established a complete system of free public health care. Hospitals, pharmacies, and other medical facilities were nationalised and handed over to the district health authorities. Departmental hospitals were created and were started in industrial enterprises and ministries for certain categories of citizens (party leaders, military and security personnel, miners, workers, heavy industry workers, transport workers, etc.)

Health care was managed by state, and funding came from state revenues under state plans of social and economic development. All health care workers were in the service of the state, which was paying them wages and ensured the supply of medical institutions. The Ministry of Health under the strict control of party leadership issued mandatory standards for medical facilities and personnel. The main focus of health policy in those years was the expansion of hospital beds and to increase the number of health professionals.

For determining the HCS typology, it is most important to agree on the formal criteria on which they depend. M. G. Field divided them based on the socio-political structure of the society and identified five types of health systems: (1) classic (disordered), (2) pluralistic, (3) insurance, (4) national, and (5) socialistic.

M. Fotaki considered the modern health care system based on different levels of social development. So these were the following models: (1) universalist (Beveridge model), (2) social insurance (Bismarck model), (3) 'southern model' (Spain, Portugal, Greece, and partly Italy), (4) institutional or social democratic 'Scandinavian model', (5) liberal (residual social security), (6) conservative corporate (Japan), (7) Latin American, (8) health care of industrialised nations of East Asia, and (9) health systems of countries with transition economics. Many classifications suggested that there was no understanding yet of the underlying causes of the various systems.

Having examined the early health care systems, it becomes apparent that for any state there is a need to solve two interrelated global problems; they look very similar but have different targets:

(1) *To provide an opportunity to conduct individual changes in the patient's body* to preserve his life, with the elimination of pathological focus to the point of being comfortable, allowing him to work as well as show some improvement in his body at a reasonable price for him.

(2) *Get the opportunity to have an advantage over other groups of individuals* competing for a economic or ecological niche; in terms of the nation state—to help the citizens of this state have biological competitive advantage over citizens of other states (live longer and be more workable). A complex of such measures as purely medical and non-medical recently is called *social policy.*

It is clear that these requirements existed before, but were not understood yet at the level of national elites because of the global economic challenge, the solution of which was that we should regularly invest in resources. If the solution of the first is simply to have modern medicine, then the solution of the second needed a specific tool—the health care system.

The archaic system of health services looks like this:

- There were no mediators between the doctor and the patient.
- Monitoring the effect of the application of medical technologies was carried out by the patient (or their relatives) at the level of 'like' or 'dislike'.
- Fees were in given in cash or real form at the time of service performed or immediately thereafter.
- Amount of compensation was determined by supply and demand in the local market by negotiation between the doctor and the customer.
- If there are no resources to pay the doctor, the service was not provided.
- Motivation to doctor for providing services was purely commercial—selling knowledge and skills.
- The above second problem was not solved in general because of the lack of motivation for both actors (doctor and patient).

After organising the aforesaid health systems, the situation changed:

- A mediator appeared between the doctor and patient (or merchant or government structure), which solved several problems:

  - *for the patient*—control over the results of the use of medical technology, monitor the adequacy of the price of the service, control over doctor's qualification;
  - *for the doctor*—to ensure solvency of the patients, there should be control over the very fact that the doctor gets paid with rational distribution of patients among doctors;
  - *for the state*—the accumulation of money to pay for medical workers in case of sudden and massive illness or injuries, in fact, insurance of the state for fulfilling their

social obligations, monitoring the validity of the material requirements of doctors, monitoring the training of doctors and the effectiveness of medical technologies in general;

- *for themselves*—a commercial return for its development as a mediator.

- The amount for their services was determined by supply and demand in the local market between a doctor and a mediator; the patient was present in the new market—insurance services market.
- Fee for service was only in currency, and, moreover, cashless.
- The service was not provided when the patient couldn't pay for the service, but when he could not buy insurance from a reseller, the probability of such an event was much less.

You can see that the early health care systems changed the system of motivations in a social sense, but in economic terms, they created an intermediary between the doctor and patient; in this case, there were both positive and negative consequences. Implications of such systems have been both economic and social (it is clear that this division is rather arbitrary) and are reflected in Table 4.

Table 4. Effects of mediator between the consumer and manufacturer of medical services

Positive	Negative
Social	
The agent-mediator was motivated to identify the most effective medical technologies and pay for only them.	Patients largely lost the freedom to choose their own doctor.
Far more people could become solvent consumers of medical technologies.	Mediator was not interested in 'closing' medical technologies. Moreover, he tended to counter them.

Accessibility in help led to a sharp reduction in deaths of people, including children. There was an increase in the average lifespan.	The agent, along with the state, was interested in reducing the number of medical consultations, contributing to chronic diseases.
The agent was interested in more doctors for more complete coverage of medical services.	
From material production off a large group of people involved in the new intermediary business—health insurance, while creating new jobs.	
The agent was interested in increasing the number of wealthy people in the area, as they were the potential customers.	
Economic	
Now it was possible to accumulate resources for the provision of health services to a large mass of people at the same time (war, natural disasters, epidemics).	The patient lost the ability to influence the final cost of medical services.
A larger number of people could receive medical services, thus increasing the market for such services. The number of economically active population as a whole increased.	There was an opportunity for monopolistic collusion between intermediaries and providers of health care services, leading to a sharp rise in prices.
Now you could invest only in medical technology with proven efficacy.	
The functions of monitoring the effectiveness of treatment were separated from the actual treatment functions. Quality control systems in medicine were established.	

Prices for medical services became available for global control and alignment within the state.	
Matchmaking and insurance services created many 'white collar' jobs in medicine and dependent markets.	

Positive effects of the appearance of mediator were quantitatively greater than the negative ones. It seemed that depending on, namely, effects prevailing in the given society, a modern observer attached the label to this HCS, which means 'type' of the system by some chosen scale. Considering the medical history of the twentieth century, the following global trends can be seen:

- Patient spending for purchase of medical services has become a routine item of expenditure and can be pre-planned.
- The number of health workers, which increased sharply to 300 last year, has stabilised in all countries. And stabilisation has occurred even where the market mechanisms of regulation of employed health care workers were disabled for various reasons.
- Doctors and nurses are increasingly involved in routine scientific work (interviews, screening the population, drug testing, etc.). The words 'health worker' and 'scientist' are increasingly being fused in the people's minds.
- Medicine is becoming more and more an industry; its research intensity is continuously increasing. In the last hundred years, medicine and health care have become essential expenditure in all countries. Advances in medicine have begun to be dependent on the degree of technological advancement of the given society.
- Medical knowledge of the population and, consequently, the level of interaction of people with medical workers is

continuously increasing; medical knowledge 'creeps' in and cannot be cast out. 'Everyone understands medicine now.'

- Instead of infectious diseases that are deemed to be eradicated, there are other, previously unknown or already known, diseases but in a new guise. And new infections are clearly more than the old ones that are missing.
- Health care systems in all countries were clearly not ready to tackle new problems that had arisen due to revolutionary advances of medicine. It looked like progress in medical technology and development of the health care system should meet each other and not overtake each other.
- Post-industrial patient was no longer seated in one place and quickly moved around the planet. To ensure that health care appeared fundamentally to be a new business, assisting companies helped patients to communicate with doctors as well as with stakeholders—insurers, and there are intermediaries between intermediaries.
- The number of nosological items according to the development of science was growing rapidly. Old and familiar common diagnoses were split into smaller and extremely specific groups. For the diagnostics, new and more new nosologies with specific treatment, more diagnostic efforts, or special equipments were required that increased the final prices for treatment.
- In the world, there was a growing community of physicians who had their own financial and production resources and had some mobility. The Red Cross set up to help the wounded and prisoners of war in the late nineteenth century was replaced by new, multinational, well-funded, and equipped organisations. They showed special performance in the provision of medical care in developing countries.
- The growth in revenue of medics which was fairly sharp in the early twentieth century almost stopped, as the financial capacity of most patients who could afford health insurance

was exhausted. There was a tendency in many patients in developed countries of a gradual transition back to the archaic forms of payment for medical care (cash for service), for which they travelled abroad (medical tourism).

To answer the question posed in the title 'Are there types of health care systems?' we must first know what determines the type of defined health care system. From the point of view of the nature of communication parameters of the environment health system, it is always *open*, which freely exchanges energy, matter, and information with the environment. Indeed, it is impossible to imagine a *closed* system of health care. By origin, it is always a socio-economic system. What is the difference between the health care systems of different countries?

In my opinion, they differ only in the manner in which they collect and accumulate funds to achieve the goals and its own maintenance. The only source of funds for the system is the money of potential customers, who are all citizens of the given country. All other levels of the system are essentially the same in all countries, the only difference being in the methods and level of motivation of participants and the number of intermediaries through which the payments go. It turns out that the diversity in health care systems in the world is in fact that it is the only possible form. Well, tell the reader which types are possible? Or, more precisely, ask what should be the difference in the types of health systems, if they still exist?

Any social system is a materialised hierarchy of values of the given society, furnished with legal limiters and stitched together with economic motivators that play the role of positive and negative connections. HCS above was defined as follows:

Health care is a way to organise life within the species, which aims to ensure its survival in the given environment and to provide the development in accordance with certain

goals that used medicine as instruments, as well as all
social institutions that were developed in a given society.

How should we imagine a hierarchy of values, individual and
collective, in modern human society? The first are physiological
needs, see Table 5.

Table 5. The hierarchy of values in modern society

Individual value system	Collective value system
The survival of an individual (instinct)	The survival of the general population
The survival of the family and closest relatives (social motivator).	Public health of the population in general (especially children)
Individual health that provides performance (economic motivator)	Balanced demographic growth of primarily the working population
Health of family members, providing efficiency and the ability to learn (economic and social motivators)	Recognition (self-recognition) of society as being successful compared to others
The need for security: the belief that payment of medical care does not lead to ruin	
The need to recognise the individual as successful	

Abraham Maslow in his *Theory of Human Motivation* (1954)
defined the basic human needs as a hierarchy of values:

1. Physiological needs: food, clothing, housing, and leisure.
2. The need for security: the need for security and stability;
   dependence; protection; freedom from fear, anxiety, and
   chaos; and need for a structure.

3. The need for belonging and love: lust for warm, friendly relations, the need for belonging to a social group that would provide him such relationships, the family that would accept him as their own.
4. Need for recognition: the need to feel your own power, efficiency, competence, self-confidence, independence, and freedom.
5. The need for self-actualisation: the desire of man for self-realisation to update is embedded in his potency. This is a need to develop intellectual abilities.

The very first physiological needs of citizens (points 1 and partly 2 by Maslow) have to deal with medicine and HCS of any state at the current stage of development. To recognise this obvious fact is to recognise that HCS is the backbone of the economy of any developed country, that it provides a workable population of the country, and that it is such a *value which the state if at all desire cannot buy with money*. So I think that the main criterion by which we can determine the type of HCS in general is exactly how well this system satisfies the above basic needs of the given society (from the first to the fifth point by Maslow.)

Types of human societies are different, but the basic needs of each are exactly the same because we are dealing here with instincts. The identity of the instincts (survival, maternal, and so on) determines the identity of the value systems of all living people, even the tribes of Equatorial Africa and the Amazon, which are living tribal systems. A logical conclusion is that in a society human beings have reached a certain stage where the HCS should be just as we observe around us, because it is forced to satisfy the base and absolutely identical human needs. Fundamentally, HCS can only be different in the following cases:

- basic human needs change, but it will be another social being and a very different society, whose pyramid of priorities will be different;
- HCS learns to satisfy the basic needs which are next in order of priority, such as point 3: 'the need for belonging and love' that is directly involved in the formation of the family in society, or learns to satisfy this need in a different way.

So the answer to the question posed in the title of this chapter is: *At the given stage of development of the human society, only one type of HCS can exist or none will exist.* In the next chapter, we will try to understand what will be the main sign of this only possible kind of HCS.

2. G. What Determines the Properties of the Health Care System?

Social systems differ from mechanical systems by one fundamental difference—they consist of living beings that have instincts and some hierarchy of needs determined by these instincts. Needs and instincts of a group of individuals form the primitive social system aimed at its survival with minimal energy losses. Configuration of the system depends on the environment, no less than the kind of most living creatures; to put it more precisely, the community of living beings interact with the environment in which it is located or produces a productive social system that allows it to survive or perish. It is important that the initial set of environmental conditions and characteristics of beings inevitably leads to only one possible type of social system. A very rough analogy: if stones are dropped one by one on a flat piece of land, you will inevitably get a pyramid; its specific configuration will depend on the magnitude of the acceleration of gravity, uniformity of sizes and shapes of stones, and the properties of the surface. If somebody does not want to obtain a pyramid, someone from 'outside' must change the initial conditions.

In case of social systems of human society, the situation is much more complicated: Each unit which consists of a system has the intelligence that sets goals and more or less free will to achieve these goals. HCS, as mentioned above, satisfies the basic individual needs of each person, as well as basic collective needs of the population as a whole. Since these requirements are the same for all people and societies that they form, then the target system, which is formed to meet such needs, will be the same. How should we describe the *properties* of such a system?

1. *Statement of purpose*: Each system can only ask themselves the following goals, by which they can see, understand, and measure the degree of achievement of and then use

this knowledge to adjust their work, creating feedback. The objectives are derived directly from the hierarchy of values of the society, which in turn is determined by the biological essence of a social being. The global goals of HCS at this stage of development are actually only two:

1.1. *Getting the competitive biological advantages by the population in comparison with its neighbours*: This includes all the smaller subordinate goals, such as treatment of medical cases, reducing the overall morbidity and mortality, improving efficiency, creating a favourable environment for yourself, collective immunity, and others. The question 'what will be a competitive advantage in these conditions for these creatures?' usually is outside the competence of the HCS.

1.2. *Getting the ability to change at will the basic properties of organisms that make up the population*, including longevity, ability to reproduce, and the period of performance.

2. *Terms goal*: Logically thinking, the planned timing goals should be less than the lifetime of the technologies that achieve these goals. If a medical technology has reached a goal (made the change) at a time when the technology itself is outdated and has been replaced by another or even abolished, its results cannot be used to adjust the technology and the system as a whole. This result is outside the system, and usually, it is not noticed in the system. In practice, it is clear that the time shift in medical technologies are increasingly shortened; that is, terms of achieving appropriate goals should decrease even faster. The question remains open: What if social technologies do not have time to develop for purely medical technologies?

3. *Means to get the goal:*

   3.1. *Creation and development of the most effective medical technology A* (or *'closing'*, i.e. those that solve medical problems for this generation or, in the ideal case, *'perfect'*, i.e. technology, the result of which is inherited): The question of efficiency of the given HCS *ceteris paribus* is likely to be dependent on the ratio used in *'imitational'*, *'intermediate'*, *'closing'*, and *'perfect'* medical technologies, in other words, from the fact that the number of medical problems of population can be solved fundamentally and forever.

   3.2. *Building on the basis of the most effective medical technologies B* and preparing qualified and motivated medical workers in sufficient quantities.

   3.3. *Changing the environment of all members of the population* or its individual target groups that promote the achievement of HCS objectives.

4. *Tools for assessing the adequacy of the results*: It is clear that every goal system aimed at the moment of its production must assume its method of recording and assessment. The absence of such an instrument is equivalent to an infinite term goal (or its failure to reach), because the system will never be able to see that goal has been already achieved.

5. *Coverage of potential customers*: Here there are many gradations of accessibility; starting from the caste system for the elite to the full availability of all the people living in the area, including the temporary population and foreign citizens. This question is not so much the number of available resources as a political choice of designers.

6. *Price of the system's functioning to the public:* This is the most prominent and debated parameter of HCS for today.

I think, various gradations of price of the system are often seen by mistake by many researchers as the various kinds of it. Rationality with which the current HCS administers the resources cannot determine its kind, just like two self-propelled devices: one of which consumes 5 litres of fuel per 100 km, while the second uses 30 litres per 100 km—both are cars. Small differences in the engine design cannot make them anything else.

If the health system was not developed naturally and was constructed artificially, the absence of at least one of the above properties of ES converts all other design into meaninglessness, social simulacrum that simulates the job, but lacks real opportunities to perform. In particular, the undelivered global goal of HCS leads to the fact that *different levels of the system begin to consider means of achieving (p. 3) as global objectives (p. 1)*; for example, the doctor of first contact starts fighting for the 'beautiful' statistics on his site, sincerely believing that this is the main sense of his work. The doctor in the regional division at this time fights for maximum turnover of beds in local hospitals; the region begins to consider increasing the number of family practicing physicians in their territory as a goal, and the doctor at the highest national level begins to consider increasing fertility as a goal. As a result, almost all efforts do not lead to the desired global results, as the effects of these goals are often directed in opposite directions.

One can also imagine the HCS which has a global goal that is *opposite* to the biological nature of social beings that the system is consisted of, trying to counteract the hierarchy of values of the given society. Such a system will spend all available resources on 're-education' of society and change the hierarchy of values as well as the biological essence of individuals, but the global goal obviously will not be achieved because we cannot change the biological nature of someone. Such a system will be self-destructed after the exhaustion of their finite resources.

HCS that puts in time to achieve some goals in the distant future may face a situation where it will not see the result achieved as tools (structure), for tracking results may become obsolete. It may also encounter a situation where the system will see the delayed results of outdated medical technologies, which no longer apply. These results of the system are not recognisable as 'their own', as there is no logical connection between technology and the result of its application. This result will be attributed to who and what you like, but do not own the work of HCS in the past.

Theoretically, one can imagine that HCS will get some results of the medical technologies more quickly than developing the means to track the results. These results will also be 'lost' by the system, as they will be received at a time when it is not waiting for them.

Questions about the means of achieving these goals are very important. Firstly, all the means employed by the HCS must not be in conflict with the hierarchy of values of the current society; it will have to be especially careful to monitor while importing medical technologies from abroad. Also, important questions are in accordance to medical technology B and habitat of the target group of individuals for which the technology is applied; at least they should not contradict each other.

The price of functioning of any HCS at a given time for each member of the community depends on a combination of parameters, such as the following:

- The total number of members of the society who support this HCS with their resources at the moment;
- Whether the system can generate and store 'in reserve' resources provided by community or whether they are forced to spend immediately;
- The number of customers who receive assistance from the HCS at a given time and hierarchy (priority sequence) of these clients;

- The degree of medical technologies' efficiency this HCS used;
- The number of resources the HCS spends not on the task, but to support itself;

HCS of developed countries, reaching the limits of their growth, stop in the qualitative development and begin to accumulate quantitative changes: the growth of infrastructure, the increase in information capacity and range of medical services, increase in the number of applied therapeutic methods and medicines produced. This accumulation mimics development, while improving some results, but does not lead to a new quality, which cannot occur without changing the basic parameters of the interaction of the system's components, a kind of *social phase transition* in which all elements of the system that accumulated enough social energy and resources in the moment (by historical standards) change the state of the environment throughout its volume, dramatically changing the basic properties of HCS and giving it new opportunities for further quantitative growth, but at a new level. The next section will attempt to predict how the next level of HCS would look.

2. H. What Will Be the Next Stage?

The fact that modern health care systems in all developed countries are close to the limit of their capabilities is already visible to the naked eye. Moreover, this limit is not so much on technological properties as it is on accessibility to the public in the broadest sense of the word. Looking at HCS from different countries and the way they were before coming to this state, you will notice that they all differ from one another in only ways to extract part of the social product of those who produce and ways to buy health services with these selected funds for as much of the population of their countries. A huge number of options, strategies, and a combination of financing methods has not yet revealed the 'magic bullet' that is a successful combination of solutions which would solve all problems at all. These problems are different.

How much exactly should be taken away from the producers of the social product? HCS needs in the future are unknown, so the state is trying to take away more resources as possible for future use. This happens even when the state is not cheating. In turn, the people cannot understand right now why they should pay for health care for generations not born yet, who as it may happen would not live in this country at all, especially if their own medical needs, judging by the results, which was paid for went from bad to worse. Reasoning about joint responsibility comes into conflict with the wall of misunderstanding between different generations and increasing globalisation, which results in that no one can understand where, which generation, and who paid what to whom.

Medical advances have led to paradoxical results: *the best medicine in the country, the lower the percentage of producers of the social product* (financiers would say a less taxable base), as well as an increase in the life expectancy over time increases the percentage of elderly—the main consumers of medical and social services. Thus, a smaller working population would require more and more funds for the maintenance of health and social services, and sooner or later collapse will occur: If the state takes money 'moderately', the existing modest means will be in blatant contradiction to current tasks, or if the state takes money strictly in accordance with the set objectives for the future growth, then sooner or later the social product manufacturers will raise a rebellion. Such a rebellion can be expressed in the form of more or less open sabotage or even escaping (we are talking about physical escape or transfer of business) to another country, where they will take less. In both cases, the financial collapse of HCS is imminent.

Another problem is that the *overall cost of health care is continuously going up,* and the rate of such growth increases nonlinearly. Those services that seemed a fantasy ten years ago now no longer satisfy anyone. Medical facilities throughout the world instead of becoming cheaper constantly become more expensive as technology progresses and entail costs of medical care in general. No one wants to use a computer scanner that is ten years old; everyone wants the latest, regardless of whether they have to put money on it. Medical technology is constantly at the front of scientific progress because everybody knows that outdated medical technology is impossible to sell. There are people who drive old cars that are twenty or thirty years old and will ride them as long as those cars are able to move. There are clients who are fond of using old things, devices, and vehicles. You surely will not die because you are wearing old clothes, listening to an old radio set, watching a black and white TV, and driving an antique car. But in medicine, such loyalty is not observed; all consumers want to use the most recent developments, since it affects the quality and duration of their lives. This is one of the rare economic behaviours of people when almost the entire mass of customers does not want to be loyal to the old brand (of course, the brands mean technology rather than individual companies.) Unfortunately, the rate of rise in the price of medical technology is moving ahead of income growth, even in developed countries. Each new discovery in medicine costs more and more in terms of investment in science, and this process is accelerated. Extrapolating the process, it is a logical finish that latest medical technologies would be available only for a few persons with the greatest revenue and scientists themselves, who would use their findings on a pilot basis. The area of availability of advanced medical technologies is shrinking like shagreen leather, and how to prevent it is not yet clear yet.

The feeling of swaying under the feet in public health finances is felt by all countries, including most developed and rich countries, the system of health insurance running until the last time—more precisely, the system of 'stretching' the umbrella of joint responsibility and solidarity risks over the maximum of population by the accumulation of premiums magically stops working. It is expressed in the fact that *less and less of medical product can be purchased for the accumulated premiums*. The collapse of the system is not far off.

Another problem that concerns HCS deepens the health care crisis and has recently appeared—globalisation of all markets, including the health care market. The paradox is that *only medical services are globalised, but not public health*, which stubbornly refuses to let go at the supranational level and leave the 'private' and unique for each country. This is quite logical, since the health systems are very much tied to the political systems of different countries (in some sense, they are a reflection of the political system); a local taxpayer spends money on their maintenance but medical service always stays out of politics and only applies to the buyer and seller. A client who is now informed of his illness and is aware of the most advanced technologies for its treatment knows where it is possible to achieve the best results. State borders are no longer an obstacle, and if he wants to be treated by a foreign doctor in a foreign hospital, there is no law forbidding that. The result is a growing export-import of medical services in the world and the free flow of capital in medicine; also, patients who come for treatment in a country actually invest their money in medicine of that country, but not in its health care system. This medicine, which receives recharge from abroad, begins to live its own life and ceases to depend on the HCS of this country. Instead, it begins to financially and ideologically depend on the global health care market that is spontaneously formed. Thus all health systems, locked in their national apartments, converted into 'holey pots' for the economies of their countries because by definition they cannot control the money of patients-taxpayers that are freely flowing across borders.

Thus, we see *two types of failure* of national health systems: In countries with advanced medicine, we see how swollen the medical field is from the 'outside' money, and in fact, medical business (regardless of the real owner) separates from its HCS and starts telling their market requirements, then public health with all its attributes slowly fades and is replaced by the board of directors of a medical mega-corporation that is more or less in a non-targeted manner using taxpayers' money of the country for the benefit of rather the international medical community (not necessarily of the given country). The second type of failure can be seen in countries with underdeveloped medicine, which cannot profitably sell produced medical services in the global market (or they are services of poor quality or they are too expensive). In such countries, the import of medical services takes place, that is, the population with enough money leaves for treatment abroad. There seems to be nothing wrong for HCS if the client initially pays for medical services in his country in the form of medical insurance or taxes and then goes abroad to pay for services once again. The crisis comes when these processes become visible by consumers, and they start sabotaging payments within the country, while the umbrella of solidarity for those who cannot go abroad for treatment becoming holey and still full of holes, and at some point, there comes the infrastructure-personnel death of the national HCS that cannot hold itself any more. It happens because HCS makes planning for the total population, but not just for poor, which cannot travel abroad for medical services and percentage of which cannot be predicted in advance. The crisis of such a system is complicated by the exodus of medical personnel who go where they are paid more, which is attached to the global health care mega-corporation that develops the global health care market.

HCS of all countries, starting its development at different times and evolving with different speeds, relying on dedicated public resources and the efficiency with which they can absorb, come to the same state where it's *impossible to keep qualitative growth, despite continually extracting resources from the community.* The situation is exacerbated by globalisation, which for HCS is expressed in that social energy in the form of dedicated resources, using a variety of mechanisms, flows freely between national borders, often completely unaware of them, which leads to the fact that all the national health systems on planet behaves like a single unit, accumulating total internal social energy. There is a very rough analogy with the *thermodynamic phase transition*:

Dynamics of phase transitions (by Wikipedia)

> Under the abrupt change in the properties of a substance refers to a jump in temperature and pressure. In reality, however, affecting the system, we do not change these values, and its volume and its complete internal energy. This change always occurs with some finite speed, which means that in order to 'cover' the entire gap in the density or specific internal energy, we need a finite time. During this time the phase transition does not occur immediately in the whole volume of substance, but gradually. In the case of first order phase transition is allocated (or take) a certain amount of energy which is called the heat of the

phase transition. In order for the phase transition did not stop, you should to continuously take (or sum) the heat or compensate it by doing the work on the system.

Thus, we can predict that while all the social energy is supplied in the form of resources that are not distributed evenly throughout the volume (in our case—among all countries on the planet), the phase transition into a new state cannot occur. Of course, we are talking about moving to a single planetary HCS. The pertinent question is: *Is a local phase transition possible?*

The answer will depend on some parameters of the social medium:

- The speed of the interaction between the regions in the volume of social 'matter': By interaction, it must be understood the exchange of population and medical technology B, the exchange of medical personnel (carriers of advanced medical technology B), the spread of a healthy lifestyle, including standards for quality of food and drinking water, information and cultural pressure of areas with greater energy in a region with lower energy. The speed of interaction also affects the ability of regions with excess social energy to 'share' it, as well as the ability of regions with low social energy to 'master' it when entering from the outside. Such skills of states are in the competence of politicians beyond the scope of this book.
- Presence of closed (inaccessible) areas inside the social 'matter': The more these closed areas (regions, countries, closed social groups) in which HCS cannot assimilate the resources coming from outside and/or prevent the commission of work on the system, the more likely that excess production in the areas of social energy local phase transition occurs. By quantity, it should not be understood as the number of such areas in pieces and the value of their

total volume with respect to the others. By unavailability, it should be understand the impossibility of sharing resources namely between HCS (as well as areas where HCS has not appeared at all), but not between the political and economic entities on the world map.

- The intensity and effectiveness of doing the 'work on the system': From the definition of phase transition logically follows that increasing the internal energy of the system can be either a continuous supply of energy from outside or commission work on the system (from the outside or inside). That is, it means that the HCS may undergo changes not only because of the uploading of resources in it but also because of work done by the information transformation. Source of transformations can be both outside and inside the system. Clearly, the idea that the system can supposedly 'warm up' itself will cause a smile in physics—the low energy conservation has not been cancelled, but the social system can manoeuvre with resources, deliberately siphoning resources from one subsystem to another, including making one of its subsystems 'work' at the expense of another.

That is, the reader is fed the idea that qualitative changes in HCS of any country can happen when the planetary HCS, which actually consists of all of the national HCS and even those areas where HCS has not been formed yet at all, more or less allocates resources and social energy throughout the scope, and then in places of concentration of social energy the local social phase transition is accomplished, which changes the basic parameters of HCS (global goals, timelines, resources, tools, and price of the system). Then the new state is gradually extended to all the available social 'matter', and only at this moment will then a new stage of quality growth for a united HCS be possible. The specific location (country) where such a transition will be fulfilled first cannot be called, because it depends on a huge number of random factors that overlap randomly.

So, let's summarise the chapter. Watching HCS of developed countries, the problems through which they cannot 'jump' with all the available current resources have become visible. Accumulating quantitative changes, these HCS are becoming more and more expensive to operate, but cannot bring decisive advantage to their owners (local taxpayers). Let's list the main problems in the most general form:

1. *The principle of insurance in the medical case is exhausting*: In contrast to accident insurance (fire, flood, robbery, etc.), health insurance has to do with the insured event, which could happen now with almost 100% probability. As possibilities of medicine and the age of the patients increase, the number of medical conditions and diseases that are recognised as insurance claims have become more and more; thereby, the work of insurance company makes less sense. Insurance premiums for citizens in such conditions actually become cumulative contributions to the treatment of disease, which certainly will follow. Trying to survive, the insurance companies are starting to invent ingenious ways to save money on the examination and treatment, a system of accumulative discounts for customers, and complex and group insurance plans, but it helps very poorly. The financial bag, which now represents the insurance companies, instead of helping to streamline and expedite payments (and it was done at the start of the health insurance system), turns into its opposite—makes the payments difficult and diverts the resources of present and future patients to the maintenance of the structure which they do not really need. The only reason for this accumulation of funds for future treatment is the bank interest on these funds, but the same can be done by the

usual bank, and the percentage will go to the perspective patient, not the insurance company. Thus, health insurance, in the form we know it, i.e. as a kind of business, exhausts its social meaning.

2. *Modern technologies increase the cost of medical procedures and treatment in general*: The more expensive is the diagnostic and treatment equipment, the more advantageous it is to produce, and the larger hospitals are interested in the speedy return of their considerable investment. Thus, it is a vicious circle: The hospital gets increasingly expensive equipment, all the time increasing the final price of the treatment for the patient to quickly get a return on their investment to buy more expensive equipment, but its producers are investing all their profits into new technology development, creating new diagnostic and treatment capabilities (often having no relation to the real needs of the patient and the physician) for their customers at a more expensive price. The coils of this 'medical arms race' are shortened, draining the wallets of patients with each loop.

3. *Globalised patient*: He is a patient who can freely move around the world and choose a hospital for treatment, and the doctor creates an unprecedented thing: the global market for medical services. A doctor in New York and a doctor in the province of Thailand (or in Egypt) will suddenly find themselves in a competitive environment, which did not count when receiving their medical degrees many years ago. Now in the global market, they have to recognise that for the patient the only meaningful outcome is the price and conditions of stay they will be able to offer. The patient is no longer worried about the prestige of the university which houses the clinic, the name of the country, its political system, and the method of taxation. All obstacles are related to the fact that the patient cannot ask

for help in another clinic or in another country because of the inability to get there, as well as linguistic, legal, and other problems, quickly fly off. Internet completes the globalisation of medical services by creating a common information space, as well as for health workers and patients.

4. *Constantly moving mass of patients leads to the change in the very principles of medical care:* The physician cannot physically observe the patient during his life, as he did in the late nineteenth and early twentieth century. The old concept of 'family doctor' ceases to have any meaning, especially in the changing lifestyle of modern families who do not all live in one house as before. But there is a new concept of a family doctor who watches his family remotely using telemedicine network technology regardless of the physical location of their patients. The concept of 'medical district' is also changing; it becomes dynamic and contingent in the area which is changing rapidly both numerically and qualitatively. Computer equipment only can keep an eye on the shifting of patients and collect statistics in such circumstances.

5. *The industrialisation of medicine:* The individual art of doctor ceases to be critical. The end result of treating a patient is increasingly dependent on the actions of a large team, its equipment with medical supplies, and information technologies. The problem is the new paradigm of training for health staff, which exists now in a professional environment with multiple centres of control and decision-making. The number of specialists makes up a team which is continually growing; moreover, it consists of experts from different countries and continents working remotely, using computer networks, and there's the need to harmonise their professional environment in the

broadest sense, including medical supplies, equipment, and standardisation of data types.

6. *Immobility of therapeutic and diagnostic tools*: In the previous paragraph, it was given that the industrialisation of medicine should result in a binding of site of medical treatment and diagnostic services at a geographical point, while heavy machinery should be concentrated in one place and should not follow the patients.

7. *Age limits of the concept of continuing medical education:* The flow of medical innovations coupled with constant innovations in related fields, electronics, information and communication technologies lead to a situation in that period of life during which modern physicians matching the concept of continuous medical education will be reduced. That is, it is impossible to imagine that all older doctors would occasionally sit down at the desk and learn fundamentally new things in their profession. The problem is that the number of physicians involved in the practical treatment in lifelong learning conditions will be gradually reduced in the younger age groups. Another thing is that the notion of 'old doctor' could change.

The mentioned problems lead to the fact that there is an 'invisible barrier' in spite of continuous build-up of resources for the development of medicine, and HCS does not detect the commensurate growth of performance of the whole system. A very similar situation was observed in the aircraft industry in the 1930s of the last century: Although the designers did increase the capacity and number of engines, no matter how improved the fuel was, as they 'licked' the contours of aircraft, they could not break the sound barrier. There was even a version that is fundamentally impossible. Everything changed after the creation of the stable and the fundamentally new jet engine. But these speeds required different frame designs especially adapted to the different aerodynamics and other materials, other pilots and other means of salvation, the other air navigation, other weapons, and stuff. In short, the supersonic aircraft in the 1950-60s had to be 'built again' from almost zero level.

Returning to the crisis of HCS in developed countries and taking into account the above rather mechanistic analogy with the history of development of supersonic aircraft, we can predict that the following:

- Further attempts to obtain fundamentally new results by increasing the percentage of the country's GDP allocated to her health were obviously hopeless. This disease cannot be cured by such simple means. It requires an *entirely new idea of financing* not only for therapeutic and diagnostic measures but also for public health interventions for the family, community, city, region, and continent.

- *Denial of medical insurance of a case as the type of business (entrepreneurship).* It seems we need to start accumulating the public funds in all the countries for future medical problems of our population. Resources not spent on treatment of previous generations should be accumulated for our children. There seems to be a requirement for offsets between the states in providing assistance for 'not their' citizens in the form of cash substitutes (virtual payment units).

- Attempts to construct the individual units of the new public health system, such as new ways of funding, new ways of training, new ways of motivating patients and others, cannot work individually and looks like an attempt to put a powerful jet engine on an old glider—wings fall off the plane even at the time of takeoff. *The whole HCS structure needs radical revision.*

- We apparently are in anticipation of the emergence of a new science that seeks to build new social structures. I propose to call it *'social engineering'*, but from experience we know that the most awkward name will take root, something like 'Socionics'. The current sociology has gained extensive experience in describing the facts of human social life, but no one has come near the practical construction of a new social reality (incompetent experiments of Russian Bolsheviks and the German National Socialists were more like a game with matches next to the refinery and with the same results). This new science will include some other sub-sciences: the psychology of large groups of the population, demography, ethology, economics (its individual sections), and some others.

- As we know, aircraft engineers' ideas have not yet led to the emergence of a radically new aircraft; that is, the old scheme of glider found empirically in the nineteenth century continues to exist as a supersonic and hypersonic aircraft that is, in fact, already a missile. This was due to the requirement of hybridity, which would require new forms of supersonic aerodynamics, but they would have to take off and land at subsonic speed. By this analogy, the *new HCS is also likely to be the hybrid*; that is, whichever social innovations would require a new HCS, in mankind social groups to which these innovations will be not acceptable or applicable always remain separate. By which criteria such groups will stand out, it is not clear yet. I guess it is the age factor, but it's very likely a fact that different groups of population will require different health care systems.

- The new system will be linked to heavy medical diagnostic techniques. The patient will not have to physically be in the same location where the diagnostic techniques and therapeutic decisions are made, perhaps, in some cases, and even in the place where the medical procedure happens. It looks like we'll speak about the *separation of means of gathering information about the patient from means of its processing, diagnosis, and making clinical (medical) decisions.* Means of therapeutic actions will also be forced to take the most mobile view. What we now call telemedicine in future it will be intrinsically the organisational core of the new HCS.

- The new system will be much more aware of the patient, regardless of its physical location. The *automated system for collecting statistics* on morbidity, therapeutic activities and their effectiveness, and data collection as well as forecasting the situation will take place in real time.

- As soon as the number of innovations in medicine and allied sciences will grow, the time that the average doctor spends on continuing his medical education will increase. Now it looks like the periodic visits of training courses, workshops, seminars, and conferences. In the new conditions, the doctors' movements to learning places will become meaningless—*all the retraining and further training will be held remotely and directly in the workplace.* There will be a new criterion for doctor's suitability; they will start to take into account not only his results but also the degree of learning capabilities, which usually decreases with age.

- *The gradual failure of the district principle of medical service.* The relationship between physician and patient who are attached to each other will get the required character of service, similar to the ISP. The end-user only knows the name of the company which he is connected with and through which it gets all incoming and outgoing data. But he is not quite interested (other than narrow specialists) through which nodes in fact his data goes through. In this sense, the medical district may be modified in the international pool of patients belonging to a particular social group and under observation of a specific physician (or a group of physicians). But how and by whom exactly the individual patient's data is processed in such circumstances the client will not be absolutely interested. Of course, there will be new criteria for the possibility of taking and removing patients from monitoring, as well as the cancelling criteria of the specific doctors' services. One can easily predict the formation of two types of such monitoring: a new 'family doctor' in the form of lifelong observation of family members by one doctor, despite the fact that the family may be physically scattered around the cities of the world, and a new 'district' doctor involved in monitoring members of a virtual social groups, even if temporary. That is, some clients of the system will be observed by several doctors at once.

- The preventive sense of the new HCS will be expressed in the fact that the *problems of patients or entire observable social groups will be fixed before the customers start complaints*. In this sense, the doctor's recommendations can take a very strange categorical form: moving to another city or country, changing the jobs, lifestyle, changing the diet, etc. It is clear that such powers shall be specified by international standards. The next step may be the construction of habitat for targeted social groups with special needs.

- *Total unification of the medical professional environment* means the communication of the patient and physician and types of data they exchange. There will be a gradual withdrawal of oral and written language as a means to describe the condition of the patient in the direction of international unified codification of all medical states, anamnestic findings, survey results, and treatment procedures. Only after that will the true electronic medical expert systems appear which will be fully integrated into the human habitat and will help the doctor or nurse in clinical decision-making and in some simple cases be the independent decision-makers.

Summary of the Second Chapter

So, in the second chapter, we saw that the history of medicine can actually be described as a history of medical technologies, starting from the *'imitational'*, more like a religious rite, to the not yet existing *'perfect'* technology that will solve a specific medical problem of mankind fundamentally and forever.

It also concluded that medicine as a branch of scientific knowledge is still heavily influenced by religious tradition, and it's highly lagging behind other disciplines. Also, the important reason for medicine's backlog is that its object of interest (human body) is protected by law; therefore, the experimental groundwork, which is used by other disciplines, in medicine is applicable with large restriction. The laws that describe the limitations and scope of activities of physicians and biologists (as opposed to other sciences) reflect the religious public morality of past centuries and constantly contradict the current needs of society and the possibilities of medical science.

The following *definition* of medical technology was given:

> *Medical technology* is a combination of knowledge, skills, techniques, and equipment that enable a qualified specialist to affect the natural development and changes of biological objects directly or indirectly, both individually and en masse, taking into account the reaction of the objects themselves and achieving goals with the greatest degree of probability. At a certain point, it becomes a tool for the health care system.

It was concluded that, historically, medicine has become the first internationally licensed profession, which for entering the market of services required not only talent, knowledge, and skills but also a formal proof of qualification issued by an authoritative institution. The arguments on the topic 'What is the medical technology?' has led us to an understanding of how the state, for whatever reasons, is hopelessly behind in medical technologies and training for implementing them in a globalised world and face a tragic choice: either to close completely for the world and observe the slow reduction and degradation of its population or allow developers of more effective medical technologies to control indirectly the quality and the number of population on its territory.

To answer the question 'What is the product of medical technology?' it was shown that the products of medical technologies aimed at the individual organism are: changes in the individual patient's body to preserve his life, the elimination of the pathological focus to the point of being comfortable, allowing him to work, and some improvement in his body. The ultimate products of medical technologies aimed at the mass changes in organisms are an advantage over other individuals competing for a given economic or ecological niche.

To answer the question 'Can they live without health care system?' the following response was given: Countries with an early health care system and undeveloped medicine now turn to the donors of the healthy population for countries with advanced health care systems. Within these undeveloped countries, the percentage of sick population is growing, firstly, because healthy people become sick and not receive adequate care, and secondly because the healthy population moves out to those countries where there is a chance of living longer, while the unhealthy population cannot do the same as countries developed in the medical sense restrict their immigration. The quality of the population inside such a country worsens very quickly (by historical standards), economic growth is slow, business becomes impossible due to the shortage of workers and customers, the markets 'collapse', the territory of the country becomes empty, after which this country ceases to exist de facto, becoming a formality at the level of representation in some international organisations.

Having considered the earliest types of HCS, it becomes clear that the state is required to address two global tasks which are interrelated and looks very similar, but have *different purposes*:

(1) *to provide an opportunity to conduct individual changes in the patient's body* to preserve his life, eliminate pathological focus to the point of being comfortable, allowing him to work, as well as show some improvement in his body at a reasonable price for it.

(2) *to be able to have an advantage over other groups of individuals:* competing for one economic or ecological niche, in terms of nation-state, to make sure that the citizens of this state had a competitive biological advantage over citizens of other states (lived longer and would be more workable). A complex of such measures (purely medical and non-medical) has been recently called *social policy.*

The answer to the question 'Are there any types of health systems?' was that at the moment the main criterion to determine the type of HCS in the general case is precisely that exactly how well this HCS satisfies the basic needs of the given society (from 1 to 5 steps on Maslow classification). It was concluded that at this stage of development of human society only one type of HCS can exist or none at all.

Properties of the health care system have been described:

1. Awareness of the problem and goal-setting.
2. Terms of goal.
3. Means of achieving the goal.
4. Tools for assessing the adequacy of the results.
5. Coverage of potential customers.
6. Price for system functioning.

An analogy was carried out with phase transitions known from thermo-dynamics, when the accumulation of quantity simulated the development, but not led to a new quality, which could not occur without changing the basic parameters of the interaction of the components of the system, a kind of social phase transition in which all elements of system accumulated enough social power simultaneously (by historical standards) and changed the state of the environment throughout its volume, dramatically changing the basic properties of HCS and giving it new opportunities for further quantitative growth, but at a new level.

In conclusion, it was postulated that a qualitative change in HCS of any country in the world can happen when the planetary HCS, which actually combines all of the national HCS and even those areas where HCS has not formed yet at all, more or less allocates resources and social energy throughout its volume, after which the local concentration of social energy accomplishes the local social phase transition at which the basic parameters of HCS will be changed (global goals, timelines, resources, tools, and cost of the system functioning). Then the new state of system will gradually extend over the entire available amount of social 'matter', and only after this, a new phase of qualitative growth of HCS will be possible.

Chapter 3

The Health Care System Grows in Breadth

In the previous chapters, an idea was raised as awareness of the humanity of medicine—it's not just the detection and treatment of patients, as well as health care is not just the organisation of workplace for doctors; this will inevitably generate new and more general goals of health care system. Moreover, the term 'health system' gets a new meaning in such circumstances. It begins to include meanings that previously either did not exist or were regarded as separate entities, not related to health care.

This section will attempt to understand the changes that will occur in the public consciousness and, therefore, in the economy during the transition to the new HCS. Also, we try to consider the new future system emerging within the old one and make some forecasts on this basis.

3. A. The New Goal Setting: Political Economy or Humanism?

As soon as the goals of development of individual groups and mankind in general become more transparent and pragmatic, attempts to define the global goals of development in any particular area of human activity begin to come close to defining the sense of life, and then the discussion leaves the professional field and is immediately transferred to the philosophers.

Without going into the philosophy unnecessarily, I have to admit that if we consider the current strategic objectives of doctors, the health care providers, government, and the patients, the inevitable conclusion is that these goals are in fact economic, namely (listed without priority), the following:

- The doctor wants to exchange his ability to meet the needs of the patient's life for the good of himself and his families.
- The doctor wants to realise his inner desire of helping his neighbour to get moral satisfaction from their work. An employee who gets moral satisfaction from his work is the best employee.
- The physician like any other worker wants to have a stable job place and social status.
- The patient wishes to be able to work then to feed himself and his family.
- The patient wishes to realise his right not to suffer physically and morally, even during illness. Physical and moral sufferings have a negative impact on his capacity as an employee.
- The patient wants to have guarantee of his ability to work in the future.
- The patient wishes to maximise his time of the ability to work and as a whole his lifetime.

- The patient wishes to avoid paying for medical services, as well as for public services for the organisation of medical care.
- The state wants to increase the general number of workable population.
- The state wants to increase the number of people in the whole of its territory, which is beneficial for its economy.
- The state wants to reduce unproductive losses of all kinds because of illness and premature deaths of citizens.

Aforesaid contradictory political and economic demands are very old; most of them came to us from another pre-industrial society, where such a thing as social security did not exist yet. In that time, these desires are met until they do not contradict the unregulated market of medical services. With the emergence of industrial society and the importance of increasing the number of workers and their concentration in one place, the market for medical services ceased to be free and began to be regulated. The state started planning their social development, and as its instrument, there was HCS, which sought ways to meet the needs of all participants in this particular market and mitigate conflicts. The main political and economic conflict between doctor and patient is that the patient wants to receive all services at the highest possible grade and free of charge, while the doctor wants to have wealth and social status for his skills and knowledge. The political point is that both patient and doctor are the citizens of the same state and should be equal in rights, and this is not discussed.

The state policy in the health care until recently was to find a way to withdraw funds from the current and future patients so that they would not notice the grade of such withdrawal (remember that the patient does not want to pay in principle), then find a way more or less to pay money justly to health workers so that patients would not notice it, because they would have a legitimate question: And *where has the state the money*? States that have managed to construct such a system believed that they have *'socialised medicine'*.

After all developed countries have registered in their constitutions the principles of humanism and the primacy of the individual over the state as the foundation of all social organisation, political considerations prevailed and began to subdue the economy. More recently, there was a time when the states that had socialised medicine widely spread their hands to take from the budget for payments to the doctors and organisers of health, and that was enough. In recent decades, it does not any longer suffice. The most common causes are listed below:

- Along with potential, 'current' patients has become more numerous.
- Morbidity of the population is growing with a complex of reasons, including its ageing.
- The number of treatable disease entities continues to grow.
- Progress in the treatment of most diseases is very modest; improvement in the results of 1-2% is considered a big success.
- There is a large number of patients with disabilities as a result of the treatment with a 'successful' outcome.
- Besides medical market, the co-developed markets appeared, which consumed the public resources, but there was almost no effect on treatment outcomes.
- The industrialisation of medicine leads to the dependence of treatment results with the use of heavy and super-expensive technologies as well as to the sharp rise of the cost of services, including the routine physical examinations and surveys.

Feeling a lack of resources for growth, the absence of radical improvements of the results, even in rich countries that are not looking funds for public health, and chronic dissatisfaction of patients at not only the exorbitant cost of treatment but also the inability of the state to organise such rational treatment lead to loosening of the implied social contract between patients, health workers, and the state. Social guarantees of developed states towards its citizens are now being sought, not sounding like '*I pay your medical bills provided that you are being treated at our doctor, but only up to a certain amount*' but as '*I will compensate your expenses to overcome any medical and social problems provided that you are a citizen of this country*'. The paradox is that the concept of medical and social problems depends strongly on the 'norm level' assumed in this society, which in turn is continuously growing. It turns out that a developed country provides political guarantees in isolation from the ongoing economic security, but still focusing on 'yesterday's' outdated conception of the norm, sincerely believing its citizens that are living 'above normal level' will not apply for the medical and social guarantees. But human nature cannot be changed—the norm level immediately builds up to the highest possible one, with the vast majority of the population beginning to consider itself in the area they needed the social guarantees. The result is that the state *always* lacks the resources to meet the medical and social appetites of citizens.

If you look at the charts of growth of health and social costs of states, we can see that they all go up, even for those that are experiencing serious economic difficulties. To see how the curve of health spending goes down is possible only in those individual cases where a total collapse of statehood happens, when it's impossible to mark up a budget or calculate its actual implementation. Such a curve that goes down really disguises an almost vertical drop. These states, more precisely, their population, gains only generous humanitarian assistance from the outside.

But among the gently rising schedules of medical costs in different countries are those where the curve of health and social spending in the last decade is going up sharply, outpacing the GDP growth of the country. They are developed states in the social sense in which political considerations and growth targets has taken precedence over its own economy. For humanistic policies, these states and their citizens are willing to pay *any* price. Why did these states at some point considered it was possible to pay the price for medical and social guarantees for its citizens that other states that had not reached this stage considered impossible? What happened to them?

I believe that in such a society that has reached some stage the *values are really changing*. The transformation of the natural environment under their own convenience was replaced by the transformation itself as the biological objects. The accumulation of material resources of a country no longer has a target of external expansion of any kind, in any case, between the developed countries. The democratically controlled society has begun to spend the accumulated resources on themselves, on repayment of social conflicts expressed in the unequal distribution of social benefits. The consumption of really needed material goods in these countries is already close to saturation. Ceasing to accumulate a meaningless number, the country has begun to invest in quality itself. It is important that the way of managing this society allows it to realise that the 'developed country at this stage' is just a group of people who have already reached the limit of investment of their labour in the surrounding inanimate nature, in any case, at the current technological level. A growing percentage of its GDP invested in the population itself, and that is shown by the above graphs.

HCS of such a country finds itself in a continuous reform in proportion to its expanding powers and, accordingly, increases the funding for these new authorities. The population, having access to the distribution of funds at all levels of budgets, has started moving from the financing of medical activity of health workers to the construction of a new integrated social environment, adapting themselves and their organisms to the current understanding of the norm. The question is: what does this particular society consider the norm and what are the priorities in the allocation of funds with the current structure of the population?

The old targeting of the former HCS, engaged mainly in the treatment of emerging diseases and the prevention of certain classes of nosologies and birth attendants, is already looking too small for the population of these countries. There is a new goal-setting, based on a much higher level of norm, involving the human body as an object of infinite improvement. A human with such a modernised body wants to get the benefits of exercise now for himself rather than for public purposes, and the question of what exactly will be the advantage in certain conditions will lie on himself. Naturally, the responsibility for the decision will be based also on himself.

Problems of all current developed nations that are consciously trying to reform their HCS are in line with the decisions of *political and economic issues*, namely, the following:

- Realising that the current financing system of HCS cannot meet the needs of all, the state represented by the elites tried to find those groups that could be *excluded from programmes of public funding* for their medical and social needs. Politics consists of the fact that such a group all the time appears, namely, the elite of society itself.
- The HCS elites are trying to increase the state funding, for they are trying to find the state structures from which such funding could be cut. Politics is that the welfare of the elite itself largely depends on state funding of these areas. Another political point is that the unfavourable environment of these countries often does not allow them to reduce, and even more so, to completely abandon funding of many of these areas, such as defence. However, if that happens, those states are in the winning position.

- Another political factor is the tendency to *transfer the increasing severity of financing HCS on private businesses*, both in terms of responsibility of individuals to ensure the health of the population (its employees) and in the form of admission of the existence of the private health sector in which some of the money for services goes into the pockets of medical providers bypassing the state. The decision to allow private providers of medical and social services is certainly political.

- One more the political point cannot be avoided: The developed state recognises the priority of personal interests over the public ones, including disposing of their own bodies and even their lives. But for the state, the bodies of citizens are not just biological objects; *they are the parents of the next generation of the population of given country*. States instinctively oppose any encroachment of citizens to dispose of their bodies and live for the most part, as soon as there are data or simply the suspicion that such mass actions will affect future generations. This is a political issue for state, a matter of life and death.

These developed countries have decided all major economic problems at the moment and along with their citizens have some extra resources. Previously such 'extra' money was just settled in banks and become speculative capital. Now those resources are invested in those medical and social problems that were previously considered intractable or irrelevant. Previously, the state did not solve these problems itself and gave their citizens the right to decide, since resources were chronically lacking. Then the state took a political decision (or rather it were the citizens themselves through their representation at different levels in the democratically controlled state who made this decision) to spend resources on themselves, just like a family acquiring all benefits necessary for healthy living; they suddenly begin to be engaged closely with their health, fitness, prosthesis of teeth and look for a good plastic surgeon, in short, to make up their bodies and improve themselves.

Of course, this does not mean that the economic problems are absent at all. Simply, they are moved to a different level of priorities below. Political slogans of the primacy of humanitarian issues written in the constitutions finally got the economic basis for implementation. What will happen to the cost of socio-medical purposes in such countries? I think that they will continue to increase until the generation of people living in these countries does not satisfy their priority health needs. Satisfaction will come when most people will not be able to improve anything in their bodies; people will just stop to notice it, like the healthy teenager does not notice his body. Will one embellishment turn into a fashion of the exterior? Any deterioration in the general economic situation to the condition that people will begin to 'feel' their bodies again will be perceived as a national catastrophe.

Summarising, we can say that for now the developed nations provide their citizens economic guarantees of health, i.e. *'we will be healthy if earn the money together'*. In the near future, developed nations and the states' associations will give their citizens the political guarantees of health, namely, *'becoming a citizen of this country (or settling in given area)—you cannot become seriously ill'*. This is a fundamental difference.

Analysing the history of medical and social services, we can see that the medical and social status of the individual has passed several stages or cycles. The first was a *family cycle*: Social guarantees extended only to the members of the family (clan or tribe). Guarantees of Stone Age looked extremely primitive (lodging for the night, section of catch, place near the fire, primitive help with injury) but, nevertheless, gave tangible advantage for members of the clan in competition with others and when dealing with natural circumstances.

The next stage was *economic* guarantees of medical and social status: This stage began when it became possible to buy medical care with money, and the advantage was no longer simply belonging to a noble family and the economic viability of the individual. The transition to this stage was very uneven and stretched in time in different people and was strongly tied to the local religious traditions. The main feature of the transition to economic stage was mass professionalisation of physicians in Europe that began in various countries about tenth to fifteenth century and continues to this day. However, in the depths of this phase there were already visible sprouts of the next one: There was a *medicalisation* of state's activity, i.e. socio-medical tasks in the area of economic activity of people became a way of organising life within states. What one could get perilously from being a professional for money became a routine duty of the state towards its citizens. Moreover, mankind increasingly came to the opinion that if the government could not organise their work so that the availability of medical and social services for citizens was not dependent on their economic viability, such state is not considered developed.

Political guarantees of health in developed countries are becoming the norm; the new cycle of development of health care has started, and we are the witnesses of this. Interestingly, the transition from economic to political guarantees is much faster than the previous transition. One can expect that the next transition will occur even faster. For which guarantees mankind will go after the *political* ones? We'll try to talk about it in the next chapter, namely, how the health care management changes during the transition from economic guarantees of health to political ones.

3. B. New Management: Who Is Managing and What's the Object of Management?

One of the faces of the general crisis of health care in the world is the crisis of health care management. Considering the failures in the management of it, you'll notice many options of these failures. The main arising issues in this case are the following:

1. Almost each country has the Ministry of Health. But no one has Ministry of Medicine. Maybe the problem is that we do not manage medicine?

2. How to plan health care services if changes in medical technologies occur every three to four years? Maybe the problem is that we are constantly trying to manage yesterday's health care and yesterday's medicine?

3. How can the public officer manage health care if he does not understand the biological basis of the processes that he manages? How many and which kinds of educations should a manager have in health care field? And what about in medicine?

4. The patient is an integral part of the health care system. Do we need to manage patients? If yes, how?

5. How to bring the global task on the lower level of executing and not to lose its meaning because of differences in managing and executing skills at different levels of the system?

6. At what level of data collection about the managed object, do we need to exclude computers and trust only a human?

7. What is the availability in modern health care and why it is so poorly controlled?

8. How to manage a system which is continuously and unpredictably changing at the moment in making managerial decisions?

9. If we put aside the cash flow management and personnel and property management, then what else can be managed in health care? And is it necessary?

10. If a manager in health care seeks good statistical indicators, is it a sign of good managing? How to distinguish the results of 'his' administration from 'not his'?

11. How to manage the processes that contradict natural? How to evaluate the results of management if they are accompanied by 'unnatural' stats?

12. How to manage the health care of one country if the outcome affects the works results of the HCS of all the neighbouring countries or, more precisely, all the countries on the planet?

Similar questions can be asked in dozens. The abundance of issues in health care suggests that we do not understand something very deep in this process. Management in other areas of human activity is much more reliable and, most importantly, has the clear results of all, because there we manage objects that are created by ourselves. In health care, this is not the case.

As mentioned in previous chapters, medical technologies give a probabilistic result. To manage a process that for some strange reason is successful only in a certain percentage of cases is a sophisticated managerial task. Also, how should we manage the process, various aspects of which are related to each other yet not known relationships and connections? In short, why is it difficult to manage health care and *why is it more and more difficult to simulate that the obtained results are namely what we expected here*? And why fifty years ago the management of health care was obviously easier?

I think that managers around the world are trying to control the HCS, the image of which exists only in their heads and is the result of their upbringing and education that took place many decades ago. The real HCS is actually not controlled because nobody can see it whole. Described in previous chapters, the lag in the development of medicine led to a backlog of management practices in medicine, in the belief that such a conservative area of human activity must be managed exactly conservatively. The recent industrialisation of medicine means that medicine is strongly pulling ahead and breaking away from its management and appears in an uncontrolled field of possibilities.

I believe that the reasons for management failures in health care is as following. With the complexity of HCS in different countries, the managers could see that all the time they had new responsibilities and controlled objects, so to speak, a *new functionality*. This new functionality is treated as either creating new management structures within the old ones and trying to manage the new processes with the same old methods, increasing the already unimaginable administrative health expenditure (sacrificing proper funding of medical functions), or giving the new facilities under the control of management of a more or less regulated market, which was more economical for the state but much less reliable, since the market began to run not as per the state will. How do we deal with new functionality of HCS?

HCS had long ago outgrown the scale, when it could be managed from a central point by one person. Or the way of management will be changed or it will completely go out of state's control and begin to execute the commands of new, another's decision-making centre, and most of the employees of the system will not even suspect that the tasks come from another source. In these circumstances, the only reliable solution I see is the formation of a new structure of HCS on the basis of *social networks*, namely, the following:

- HCS should go to a next level and include by definition all the social functions of the state relating to health care.
- HCS should better consist of equal functional elements that are controlled by competing for the number of healthy

people serving on its territory. Resource that attract people is a new quality of public health, which can be measured. Resources of HCS can move freely between the elements by their agreement and with a specific procedure.

- Managerial global task is posed by the state in the explicitly and open form accessible to all population. All tasks should be prioritised for the implementation and have the 'value/points of success'. The successful solution of some problem should have a consequence in the form of the right of element to take the additional population to service and thus have additional income and resources. Failure in the performance of tasks should be fined by diverting some of the population of this element of the service. Success and failure should be clear and have measurable indicators.

- The client of HCS is the entire population (permanent and temporary), which is not the 'served contingent,' but a full-fledged participant of the process. They evaluate the results of each functional element of HCS and are involved in the decision-making on the reallocation of resources in the system from the worst elements to the best. Thus, starts an evolutionary mechanism for HCS elements that allow them to screen out.

- Information about the achieved results (positive or negative) should be immediately available for all other elements of the system.

- Such an HCS has no common command centre, which could be possible to deprive the funds, to isolate or to get to 'work under control,' respectively, and there is no central budget. Each element achieves a global goal using all ways and means legally available to him.

- Such HCS has a primary and a backup data centre for collecting and reporting data, where each participant of the process can see all the results of all system elements and summary statistics. Situation should be forecasted here in real time using the whole collected data. In accordance with the data presented here, the government decides which elements of the system complied with the global tasks and with which means. According to the presented data, the society through their representatives has to decide which of the elements has done the global task successfully and by what means.

- All customers are divided into sectors of 'interests' (mostly based on gender, age, and partly professional), and the system organises services for customers according to their interests.
- Elements of the system periodically check/audit each other's work on random basis according to the technique well known in advance. For each detected flaw, the finder gets the points.

The meaning of such a social network is that *it does not require administrative apparatus* of the central and intermediate levels; all global tasks can be seen all at once on the 'bulletin board' with their priorities and values. Each element of the system knows what it will receive, whether the problem will be solved, and what happens in case of failure. Each element of the system performs the task using its own resources and not begging for them in the centre. Simple and clear rules make all the elements equal competitors for the declared global values and at the same time for values for their clients, which the clients determine themselves. Competing in such a system takes place provided that the *elements of the system exist in an amount obviously greater than necessary to meet the medical and social needs* of the existing population, for which there must be some mechanism. Each new generation of trained health workers as well as health care workers who enter from the 'outside' are the 'fuel' from which new HCS elements continuously form, which come into competition with the old ones. Simultaneously, the process of exclusion of elements that could not withstand competition for the customer goes on.

Thus, the new functionality of HCS that appears either in the formulation by the population of its new public health and social care needs or when the new technical capabilities appear to meet the old needs is processed by the system at the grassroots level of the elements and does not fall to the state level. More precisely, it gets there only when it begins to influence the global health agenda of the current state.

The reader may ask, 'So what? The national health ministry in such conditions can be generally cancelled'. Of course not, but they will be quite small and their task completely changed. They will deal with the organisation of medical and social assistance for the population or some social groups that have come in unusual circumstances, not covered by standard health care protocols, and also choose from the most efficient available medical technologies and approve them as recommended for use by all elements of health systems in certain sectors. Also, they will solve tasks to standardise requirements for health workers at all levels and their qualifications. Actually, the task of the ministry will be to develop rules of the game for all elements of the system, but the ministry itself cannot be a player. Such a system is much *safer* because any attempt of corruption to take control of the centre is meaningless, since the centre does not spread any, but only recommends technologies to use. The work on the coordination of clinical work occurs only in exceptional situations and may not be a reliable source of income for corrupt officials. Attempts to take control at the grassroots elements of the system are economically feasible because it does not give a tangible benefit due to the smallness and multiplicity of these elements. In addition, this situation will be detected and eliminated during the next audit of another HCS element, defined in random order.

The meaning of such an administration is not to try and follow the actions of each element of HCS; moreover, such a task will be performed by much more interested customers of system and in the *open formulation of the global task* (the final destination point for this stage of development) that are perceived as providers of medical and social services and their clients. Performance evaluation of each element of HCS and the whole system is done on both individual customers and society on an equal basis. The sense is that all elements that are free to choose a legitimate means to achieve the stated goal will choose the shortest and most efficient way, while the remaining elements immediately pick up this decision, because it will be immediately visible to everyone.

One of the most visible drawbacks of such an HCS, organised as a social network, is an inability to fund itself for some time after its introduction due to the fact that customers must first save money on personal medical accounts before the start of functioning. That is, the implementing of such a system requires a long transition period for the accumulation of funds in which clients are fully or partially supported by the HCS of another type.

An urgent task starts to move from process management in health care to the management of actual results (and final milestones). A manager regardless of his level in the new conditions should be much freer in the choice of management methods, motivations, and strategies, guided by the principle: the completeness and speed to achieve the desired results. As soon as in the hands of medical and social services, there are increasingly powerful tools for achieving our goals, we'll need better planning; that agreed, the number of large and small processes goes up at different speeds and in different social groups. In such circumstances, a professional health care manager is the person that directly determines the image of the future population, its physical and psycho-emotional view. This is an entirely new level of responsibility, mainly future generations. Moreover, the mechanism of such a responsibility does not exist yet; to create it, it is a future legal challenge. A practical health care professional in such circumstances becomes a virtual assembly line worker, on which the entire population of the country moves (including the health professionals themselves), and as they grow older, they are converted in accordance with the plan that is worked out. The main question is the availability and quality of such a plan, as well as in accordance of the majority of the population with this plan.

From the attitudes to their own and others' health will be given to the population since the childhood depends on almost everything in society. I mean the motivation to maintain health, and consequently, the average length of productive life, the value of human life and health, and therefore the moral maxims of the society, issued in the form of laws, fertility behaviour of the population, and solving demographic problems. Demographic problems will be discussed in the next section.

3. C. The New Structure of Population: What's the New Role of Medics?

The growing demographic problems in developed countries have been marked for many years by all the specialists. These same experts say that the situation is not highly dependent on the geographic location, as well as racial and ethnic issues. It seems that matters only change the fertile behaviour of the population, which in turn is a function of production mode and the degree of urbanisation of the population of some countries and their conglomerates.

In connection with the above, the following questions arise:

1. Does the demographic problems of developed countries depend on the existence of HCS, and how are we to measure this effect, if any?
2. Is there a connection between the emergence of modern HCS in economically developed countries and demographic problems that have begun namely in these countries?
3. Will this problem spread to the entire population of the Earth, and if so, how soon?
4. How will the structure of the population in developed countries change and what will the consequences for local and global health care?
5. Which medical technologies (existing or prospective) may be used by HCS to compensate the demographic imbalances?

In human societies (populations) where any methodical medical aid is generally absent as well as HCS (usually, it is the pre-industrial non-urbanised society without any pension system), the population pyramid looks like this (Fig. 3C.1):

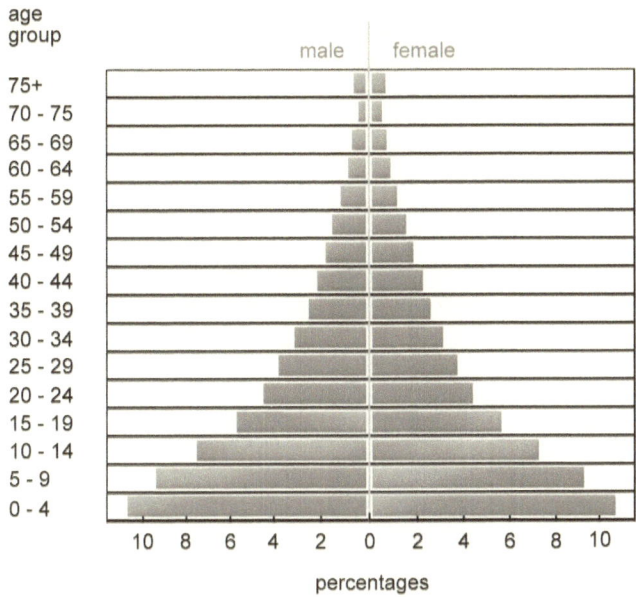

**Fig. 3C.1. The typical primitive view of population pyramid.
First stage: there is no expansion.**

Demographers call this type of population pyramid *primitive*. Such a society is characterised by high fertility and, simultaneously, a high mortality rate, at which only half the number of births survive to reach adulthood. That is, in a society there is a very high percentage of children, but only about 50% of them have a chance to become parents themselves. A very small percentage of the population survives to reach old age, as is evident from the sharpened top of the pyramid.

According to the excavation of burials in England and Germany before 3000 BC, it was observed that nearly half of the children did not survive to reach three years. In all the countries not affected by civilisation at all times or 300,000 years ago or 3,000 years ago, pattern repeats. Pyramid has a very characteristic smooth parabola concave side, and the shape of the pyramid does not change with time; if that population is not affected, social upheavals are accompanied by high mortality rates. This is the natural look of a demographic pyramid in a society where an effective system of health care is not yet developed and there no pension system.

Where does this parabolic concavity on the sides come from? We can assume that around the middle of the pyramid the natural process cease to act with the same force and the elderly who manage to live to this age begin to receive help from their older children (living pension), which slightly increases their lifespans; then there are some lucky ones who survive adulthood to see their grandchildren and get much more help—this is the steeple of the pyramid. In today's world, such a typical pyramid is found in, for example, Palestinian society (Fig. 3C.2).

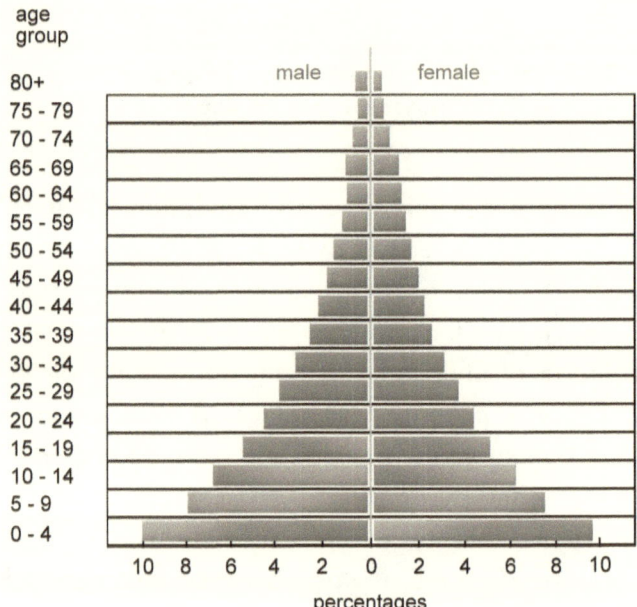

Fig.3C.2. Demographic pyramid of Palestinian society.
(*Source*: **UN Economic and Social Commission for Western Asia, Demographic and Related Socio-Economic Data Sheets for Countries of ESCWA, as assessed in 1996, No. 9 (1997).)**

It is noticeable, which is familiar to our eyes, that a significant bias to the right (feminine) side is almost absent; it slightly appears in the later years of life. I think that this case is a clear proof of how negative attitudes to alcohol and other drugs or their inaccessibility affects the shape of the demographic pyramid: In case of the hard rejection of these social vices, the form of pyramid takes a natural shape with equal chances of longevity for both sexes.

Exactly the same typical shaped pyramids are now in other countries in pre-industrial non-urbanised society (Fig. 3C.3).

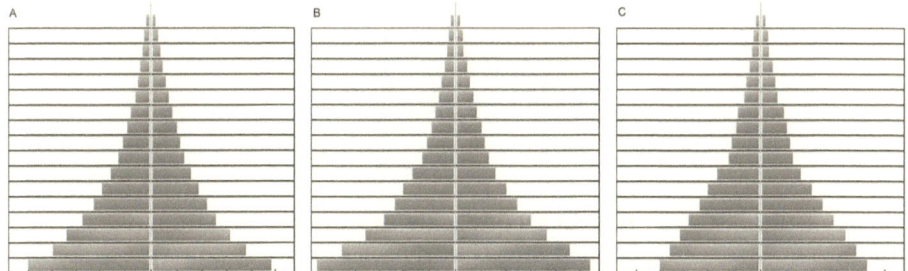

Fig. 3C.3. (a) Angola 2005, (b) Cameroon 2006, (c) Burundi 2005. Data from Wikipedia.

When such a non-urbanised society begins to seriously struggle with child mortality and starts with relatively easy things: anti-epidemic preventive measures and vaccinations, the form of pyramid changes very fast; the concave sides are smoothed out in front of those ages (demographers say 'cohorts'), which has spread with the effects of struggle with prominent causes of mortality in such a society—epidemics and famine. Concavities on the pyramid are reduced, and it becomes, so to speak, 'swell' and becomes geometrically correct.

If such actions are constant, the population pyramid comes in a steady state of early expansion (Fig. 3C.4):

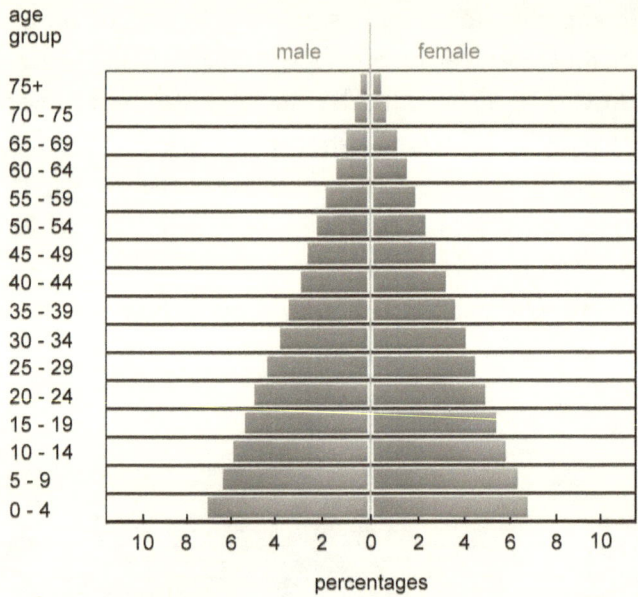

Fig. 3C.4. A typical steady view of population pyramid. Second stage, early expansion.

Mortality and fertility in such a society are still pretty high, but distributed across cohorts much more evenly than is observed in nature. Pyramid as a whole has a lower base (decreased fertility) and high altitude (increased life expectancy). Such effects have the presence of even immature HCS that the main forces have to spend on fairly simple and relatively inexpensive anti-epidemic measures. For illustration, we can see the pyramids of the following states (Fig. 3C.5):

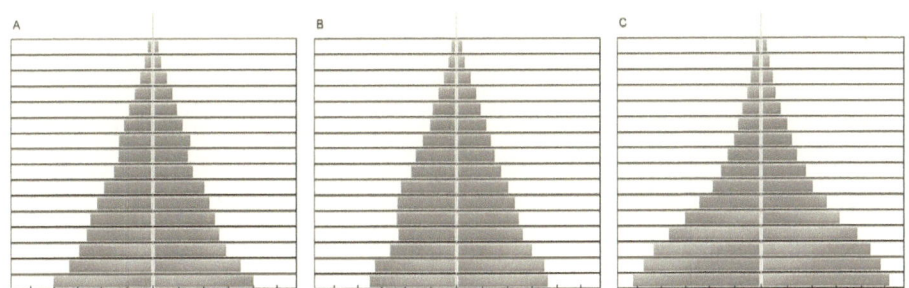

Fig. 3C.5. (a) Sierra Leone 2000, (b) Canada 1917, (c) Philippines 1997. Data from Wikipedia, www12.statcan.ca.

In some developed countries, there was a *baby boom* (a sharp increase in fertility), which happened after World War II. In this case, the typical bell appeared with sharp edges at the bottom. Here is the population pyramid of Canada in 1958 (Fig. 3C.6).

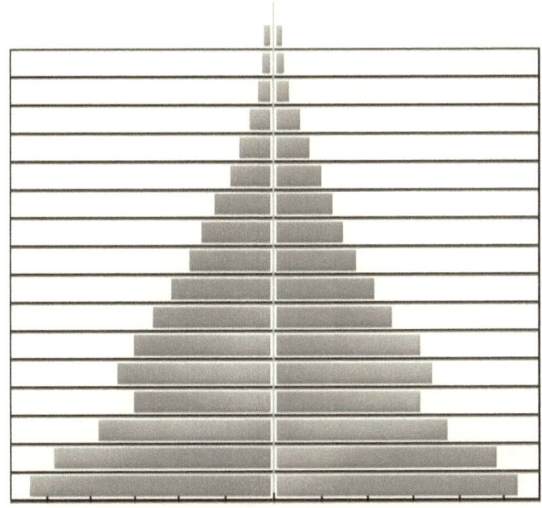

Fig. 3C.6. Canada 1958, data from www12.statcan.ca. Baby boom on the population pyramid.

Almost all countries in their development were at the given stage. The main conditions were a non-urbanised society, an unsteady pension system, and an earlier health care system occupied by the suppression of mortality from infectious diseases. But the process of expansion does not stop there: It begins urbanisation, gets to his feet with the pension system, and the average lifespan is lengthened more. The health care system, saving money for the treatment of infectious patients (no more epidemics), moves the resources and begins to fight with other causes of death, not only of children but also people of all ages. At this point, the urbanised population, which does not need a 'living pension' in the form of numerous children, dramatically changes their fertility behaviour. There is a more or less sharp decline in fertility, which is a marker of the beginning of the third stage of *demographic transition*. Also, the public awareness of the limits of expansion in the form of limited resources for growth and massive involvement in career women of childbearing age leads to depression of the fertility level. The population pyramid takes the form of a bell; its edges curves inward (Fig. 3C.7).

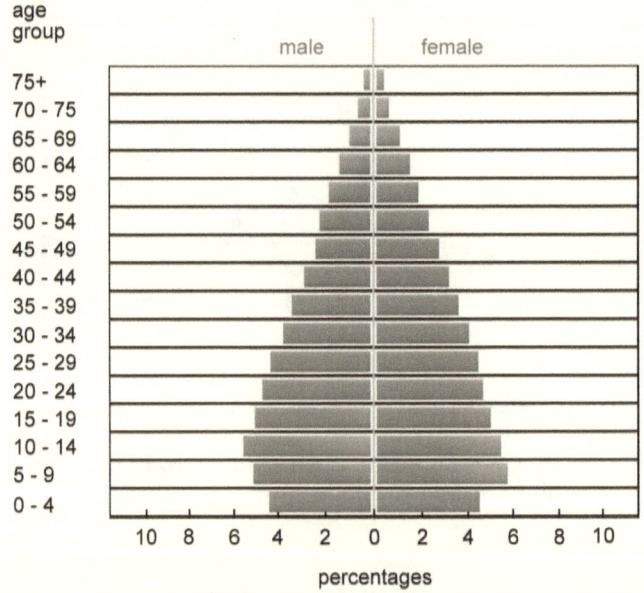

**Fig. 3C.7. A typical steady view of population pyramid.
Third stage, the peak of expansion.**

For illustration, we can see the pyramids of the following states (Fig. 3C.8).

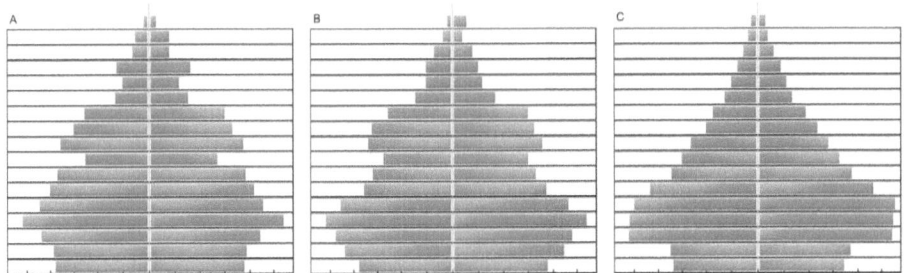

Fig. 3C.8. (a) Kazakhstan 2005, (b) Albania 2005, (c) Algeria, 2005. Data from Wikipedia.

If this situation continues for many years, the pyramid takes the shape, as often described in literature, of the 'funeral urn,' in which the new small-numbered generations form a 'foot' of urn and more numbered generations gradually move upwards.

The real problems begin at the time when the new small-numbered generations are able to work: It happens when there is shortage of workers. Such a country becomes the recipient of population (migration) from countries where there is an excess of population. The pyramid at this moment looks like this (Fig. 3C.9).

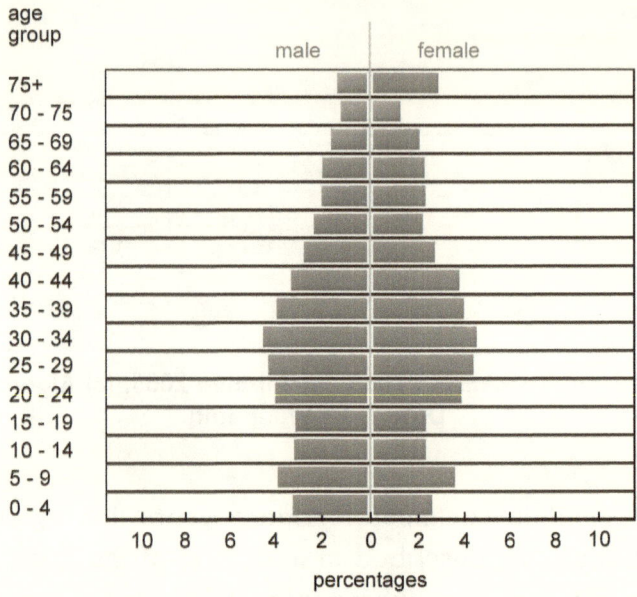

**Fig. 3C.9. A typical steady view of population pyramid.
Fourth stage, the end of expansion, depopulation.**

The extended tip of the pyramid can cause some confusion. In fact, the last age cohort in the study includes all those who are older than seventy-five years because of savings, so the top sometimes looks extended. For illustration, we can see the pyramids of following countries (Fig. 3C.10).

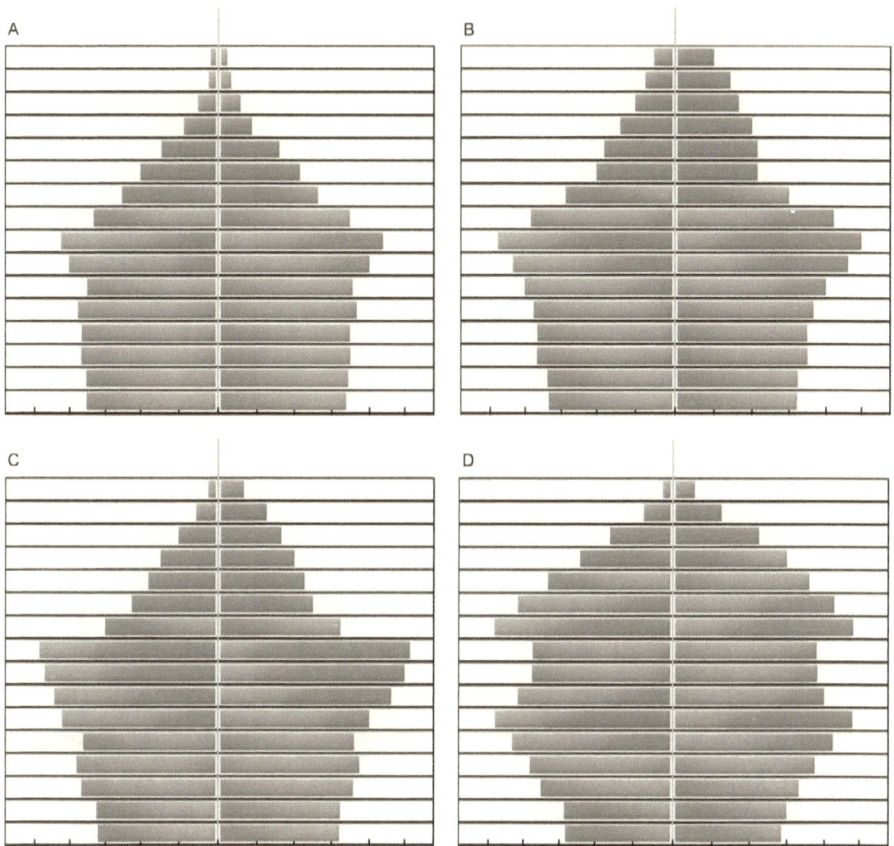

Fig. 3C.10. (a) Australia 2009, (b) Belgium 2005, (c) Finland 2005, (d) Japan 2003. Data from Wikipedia.

Increased independence and education level of women is recognised by many authors as the main factor for reducing fertility. Increasing women's education in turn leads to an increase in their independence, and the circle closes. Since the main burden of nursing and child rearing falls on women, they cannot be objectively interested in having many children.

If we imagine the future of this pyramid, it is easy to understand the level of problems to be faced by a society in the future. For example, the demographic forecast for Japan in 2050 is as follows (Fig. 3C.11).

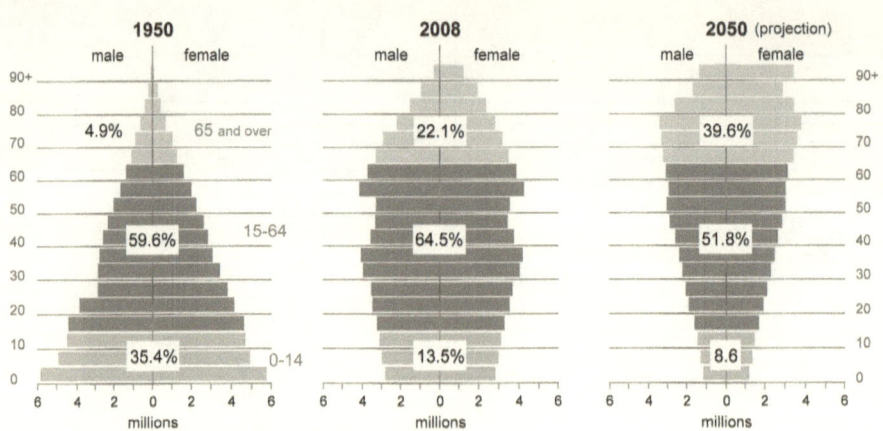

Fig. 3C.11. Japan 1950, 2008, 2050 (projected).
(*Source*: Statistics Bureau, MIC; Ministry of Health, Labour and Welface.)

It is easy to see that in 2050 52% of the working age would account for 48% of the disabled (40% of the elderly plus 8% of children). It should be noted that the able-bodied should be subtracted from those who do not produce the product: housewives, army and intelligence services, prisoners. All medical and social assistance will also be provided as these 52% of the population. It is logical to assume that the society will face a severe shortage of workers in general and social and health workers in particular. In 1950, the elderly were 5%; in 2050, it will be 40%. An eightfold increase in 100 years for essentially the same medical technologies that are not yet subjected to robotics and at the same means of social protection! After a couple of decades (in 2070), the situation will become even worse: The capacity to work will have smaller age cohorts. According to estimates, about 2050, the leader in population will be India, where 1.7 billion people would be staying. It will overtake China, which is now in first place, the forecast of which for 2050 is 1.4 billion people. In third place should be the United States, where the population would be about 440 million people. In Fig. 3C.12, the forecast shows the ratio of elderly to all others in UK until

2031. For all its territories, the explosive growth rate of elderly people in the second half of twentieth of the twenty-first century is forecasted, i.e. after ten years. Presumably, the same trend would be observed in all economically developed countries, but it will be seen in more benign forms in less developed countries. Quality of medical and social assistance to all the limited number of needy economically active population at the current level of assistance and automation technologies will simply be impossible! What should be done?

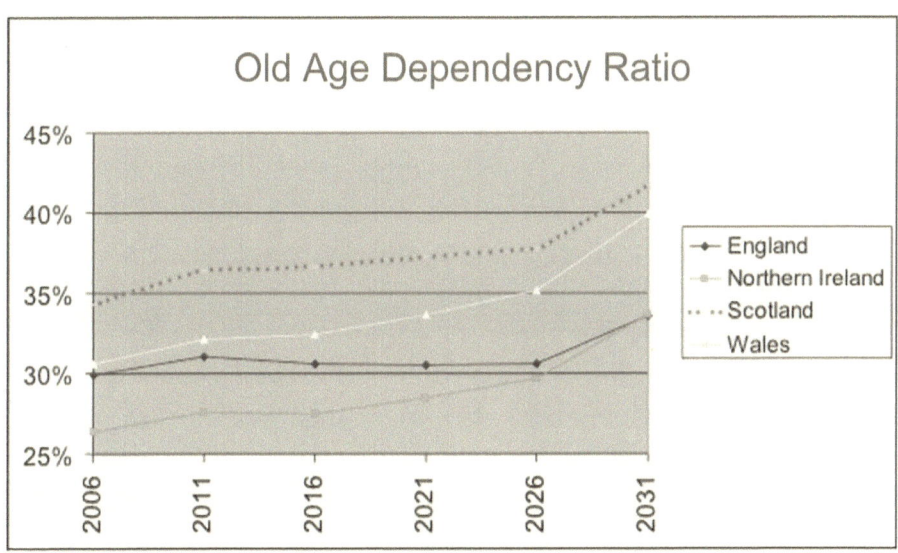

Fig. 3C.12. United Kingdom, forecast of the number of older people to 2031. (*Source*: ONS, SNPP, June 2008.)

To answer the first question 'How does the mature HCS affect the demographic situation?' we need to recognise if the system was not there (or would suddenly disappear), the situation would quickly became catastrophic. The infant mortality within one generation would return to its natural level of about 50%, with most one-child families being left without any offspring, which would just undercut the genetic diversity of population. That is a demographic pyramid of the society through a couple of generations would become a narrow column, whose height would gradually decrease over the years. In general, we can say that for countries that are in stage 4 of the demographic transition (depopulation) and have demographic pyramid in the form of a funeral urn, an effective HCS is a matter of physical survival.

To measure the impact of HCS on a society that has undergone the demographic transition is an intricate task. There are many difficulties, but the most important are the criteria of measure and the effective control group. You can offer additional years of life as an integral criterion, thanks to doctors and social workers, living representative of the average age cohort that has still the same ALE and its growth. More troubles may take place with the control group: It is necessary to exactly examine the same society with the same age cohorts, but without the HCS, and these two societies should not be connected. To get the above is possible only in conditions of direct long-term experiment, which of course is impossible in reality.

The question 'Is there a connection between the emergence of modern HCS in economically developed countries and demographic problems have begun in these countries?' is very important, because it makes us look closely at the consequences of today and especially tomorrow's HCS. To what degree the altered behaviour of large masses of people in developed countries has changed is the direct or indirect result of the activity of medical staff. Fertility behaviour of the population may be affected by various factors, including the following:

- Each family in the developed world today knows that the born child is not just the heir to the property and assets of the genus, but it is also the object of close attention of the state, which requires a soldier, student, professional, taxpayer, and parent of future generations. The value of every child in this society has increased dramatically, and subconsciously parents begin to bargain with the state for the number of their children, which makes the unborn child *product* which satisfies certain interests of the state and has a price, which fluctuates depending on supply and demand in a very specific market. How should we artificially increase the price of the goods in the market? Each seller knows the answer: It is necessary to reduce the amount, and with constant demand the price increases. So the population of developed countries does minimise the number of their children, subconsciously hoping for some preferences from the state for each of the remaining children.

- *Socio-medical services for the elderly, including pension system, become a factor that depresses the birth rate.* The state has a choice, which recently (about the middle of twentieth century) was simply not there: Where should one direct resources? To support children or the elderly? With all the blasphemy regarding this issue, it has almost always been solved by all the state officials, distributing budgets of different levels, and if you ignore it, controversy will only increase with the elderly growth rate. There is a continuous competition for limited resources of the state, and the elderly are clearly winning. Moreover, the elite of each country mainly consists precisely of representatives of this age cohort, who are quite democratically, by a majority, reallocated the resources to their advantage.

- 'Price of child' has risen sharply over the last century. The price of child now consists of cost women undergoing the labour process during pregnancy, the cost of special food for pregnant women, the cost of medical support during pregnancy, childbirth cost, the cost of patronage, the cost of newborn's 'layette', of women from the labour process during postnatal leave, the cost of vaccination and treatment of the child, the cost of his primary, secondary, and high education, the cost of his rest and recovery, the cost of his personal belongings as he grows older. Some of these costs fall on the family; some of them pay the state from taxes paid, including the same family. Note that the most significant costs for a child include costs in health care and education. Even some hundred years ago, there were such huge expenses for the child; moreover, a child that grew up in a family often helped in business and caring for younger children. Children of assistants became a burden for adults. Value-benefit currently oscillates not in favour of large families, confirming what can be observed in demographic reports of developed countries. The more developed the society becomes in terms of health and education, the more is the increase in the average price to bring the child to a working age and the more expensive becomes each 'product'. In contrast, the more 'illiterate' and medically undeveloped the society, the more 'cheap' children they can afford to produce.

- Biologists have long noticed that with the growth of the number of offspring in the population of the area, the birth rate from generation to generation begins to decline. The mechanism of the phenomenon is not known exactly, but there is no reason that in the human population this mechanism did not exist. My guess is that that there is artificial density during education of children (kindergartens, schools, colleges) despite the fact that fertility though really small leads to the fact that the whole of this generation in childhood gives a false impression of its multiplicity, and the psychological setting that it inhibits fertility in this generation remains in their lives. As endorsement, I can point to the fact that the beginning of fertility decline came in the very first generation, which in childhood first experienced crowding in education and training (transition of developed countries to compulsory secondary education). Since then, crowding of children only increased, as working adults tried to lose their upbringing and education to the state.

We can say that the very start of the process of demographic transition in developed countries has been as a result of the set of interrelated factors, one of which was the impact of intervention of early HCS in natural processes in the form of massive anti-epidemic measures—improvement of sanitation and nutrition quality. Dramatically suppressing child and adult mortality, the society over time met with problems for which it was not prepared socially or economically or technologically (in the broadest sense of the word). Their solution in the near future will probably need very different attitudes of society, until there are legislative changes in fertile behaviour and revision, rather much more clearly defining the meaning of the term 'humanity' which is pretty vague for now. After the child and adult mortality was dramatically suppressed, such a society over time encountered problems which it was not prepared to face, socially or economically or technologically (in the broadest sense of the word).

Regarding the speed of propagation of these processes to the entire population of the Earth, it can be said that there is already an increase in the speed of demographic transition in some very fast-developing countries, while after phase 2 of the demographic transition (early expansion), phase 4 (depopulation) begins immediately. An important role in these processes is an intensive exchange of young mobile population, while the new fertile behaviour occurs even in societies in which it logically could not have happened, based on the level of development of such a society. These processes of alignment have a good chance to end during the lifetime of the current globalised generation.

Demographic pyramids and population structure of countries in the context of globalisation acquire a strange appearance—mutual migration will affect the structure of society even more than mortality and fertility. In this case, in countries that are developed in the medical (and, hence, technological) sense, an 'extra' alien population will begin to appear, which will seek to live where it has a chance to live longer and better. Imbalances can occur by age and sex in large countries, even in individual administrative areas, and are so prominent that it will require state intervention to compensate them. Intervention may lie in the fact that people arriving will not just take, but gradually settle in the host country with regard to age, sex, and professional qualities. On the other hand, countries underdeveloped in medical sense would lose their populations, while their demographic pyramids will 'lose weight' and namely from the bottom, i.e. due to the young and able-bodied population, which will seek to bring out themselves and its offspring from the unfavourable environment. 'Collapse' of the economy of these countries due to lack of manpower acquires an epidemic character. There will be typical forms of the demographic pyramid for the 'host' countries and for the countries that lose its population. Developed countries will face a choice:

- to add a tough filter for the incoming migrants by introducing quotas according to age, sex, and occupational cohorts, thus giving time to manoeuvre for its HCS to adapt to taking additional clients, because the currently available resources will inevitably have to divide between its own and alien population.
- to legally deprive the new arriving population from the main advantages of using HCS, leaving them to the bare minimum until a new population will accumulate and give the resources to HCS of the host country proportionally to their quantity.
- if the previous two options will not involved, then the host HCS will inevitably divide their resources among all. Then it will quickly cease to have the resources to manoeuvre, and after a while when its growth potential is reached, the quality of services will fall dramatically and then disappear, meaning medical emigration to such a country.

Local health care systems in countries that are rapidly losing the population will experience a severe shortage of health resources, especially human resources, because the young and able-bodied medics will leave primarily. Also, it will play a role the reducing of the productive age of medical providers through the rapid renovation of medical technologies and inability to master them in old age. Other senior physicians who for various reasons are unable to leave will serve the rapidly ageing and declining population of these countries as long as the territory of these countries does not turn into a wasteland.

In global health care, in addition to routine globalisation, the processes of delegation of certain functions of national HCS at higher levels may begin, as well as separating services and sectors of activity, which did not exist at all in the local HCS. In particular, they may begin to give shape to supranational medical 'rapid reaction force' for emergency health care to be provided to the population of regions in distress, a kind of ambulance for administrative areas and entire countries, where health systems collapse (for any reason) and does not even cope well with the routine tasks of combating with epidemics and sanitary control. You can also predict the emergence of structures that govern the process of harmonisation and standardisation of medical data sharing, selection and distribution of health workers across countries and continents (something like planetary HR-departments of health system), and organisations that develop standards of medical education in the world. With the expansion of such functions and adherence to all new members, they found that this activity required a separate funding as donations to NGOs and volunteer for work for such costs will not enough. And then appeared a global health organisation with therapeutic functions (currently known as WHO does not have therapeutic functions) with its medical institutions and with their own funding, most likely in the form of contributions of joined countries. It is possible that future migration relations between states will become another aspect—health care, and that every country that lets the emigrant pay some amount to the host country for his medical and social adaptation to the new society.

And finally, the most difficult question: Which medical technologies (existing or prospective) can be used by HCS to compensate demographic imbalances? Looking at the current situation, we must recognise that the issue is not so much the availability of technology, but in particular, the readiness of society to apply them. Legal and religious constraints in biomedical technology are precisely directed primarily against the use of methods that one way or another interfere with the painful question of conception, birth, and deaths; that are precisely the issues that may influence the demographic situation. The main obstacles for the correction of demographic imbalances according to age and sex in the developed countries are not in the laboratories of doctors but in lawyers' offices and national constitutional courts, i.e. in the public consciousness. Thus, the question can be reformulated as: Which medical and social technologies would rationally be allowed to be used in countries with demographic problems?

Increasing fertility is a critical task that can lay the foundation for the future, providing it with working hands. Of course, the doctor cannot persuade or compel a woman to get pregnant if she does not want it. That is, increasing the number of those wishing to become pregnant is not at the mercy of the doctor. His power is only to ensure the right to maternity for women who are deprived of it because of natural causes or as a result of the disease:

- Treatment of female and male infertility. A complex of purely medical measures.
- Applying the technology of artificial insemination in those who cannot conceive naturally. In many developed countries, these technologies are already allowed, but usually not among the services covered by insurance or they are covered only by a limited number of attempts.

- Converting the usual pregnancy into multiple pregnancies at the request of the family when performing artificial insemination. Apparently, a special permit is not required, because anybody's civil or property rights will not be violated.
- *In vitro* fertilisation by replanting a live embryo in a healthy woman (surrogate motherhood). In some countries, it has already been allowed.
- Reducing foetal mortality and neonatal mortality. A complex of purely medical measures.
- Fertilisation of previously excluded eggs with sperm obtained beforehand followed growing the embryo in an artificial womb. They were children who by definition had no parents, except the state (the so-called 'state children'). The technology is possible, repeatedly described in science fiction, but until now such work is prohibited. Modern technology can simulate everything: foetal position in the uterus and its change with time in a day, movement and physical activity of 'mother', hormone levels during pregnancy, lights and sounds. You can even simulate the passage of the foetus through the birth canal. The question is: Is all of this enough for appearing as a healthy baby and whether state is ready for the social consequences of mass occurrence of such people? All of these children would be needed to be prepared for the surrogate family for normal emotional and sexual development, who would provide them with everything like a child born in the normal way and prepare for them places in educational institutions of all kinds. Can the state alone bear the burden of bringing up children until they are of working age, without the help of its citizens? Who exactly will determine quotas for the emergence of such children, their gender, and racial composition? Do we need to legally ensure secrecy of origin to avoid discrimination against them?

- Technology of 'liberating women from pregnancy': It is the hypothetical technology that replaces the 'social' and, in some cases, 'medical' abortion, with the prospect of its complete exclusion from practice. It consists of removing the embryo or foetus at any stage of development of the pregnancy from the uterus and transferring it in an artificial environment for maturation. This will save the majority of infants that are now lost through abortion or injuries to the mother. Similarly, it will save the life of the foetus at any stage of development in case of the mother's death. The social implications of this technology will be much more humane than a total ban on abortion or full resolution of abortion because any woman can 'abandon pregnancy' without abandoning the child. This technology will dramatically reduce the intrauterine mortality in miscarriage. Apparently, a special permit is not required, because anybody's civil or property rights will not be violated.

The state, in turn, can affect fertility indirectly through social arrangements:

- Reduction of the 'price of the child' for the family. It should focus on young parents, single mothers, women who for a long time could not get pregnant, and large families.
- The set of measures to reduce the level of substances that could damage the foetus in the body of a pregnant woman. Primarily, they are narcotic drugs (including alcohol and nicotine), as well as domestic and industrial toxins, cosmetics, and food supplements.
- Legislate the percentage of budget allocated solely to support measures to stimulate the birth rate, as the protected article of budgets of all levels.
- Recognition of the mother of many children as a self-employed citizen, with all its consequences: trade

union, pension from the state once she reaches a certain age, surcharges for additional children (more than the average number in the country), state insurance, other benefits, and bonuses.
- Counterwork of 'social' abortions. A complex of social and legal measures.

Extension of productive life is a task which allows the public to have a reserve of workers. Modern medicine has extended life up to 75-80 years in developed countries, but the sense is that the old man has lived a full life and was workable as long as possible. Performing this task in the future may help solve critical economic and social problems—the rejection of a unified retirement age and the transition to group and individual retirement ages, which will save a lot of money for social purposes.

3. D. The New Competition: What's the Goal? Rereading of Michael Porter

In any field of human endeavour, the major motivators are adversarial, with an unwillingness to be lagging, and the activity of medical providers is no exception. For what actually do the medical providers compete and patients and how will this change in the future? It is convenient to consider the example of USA as competition in medicine, which has a medical market in its purest form.

I must say that the U.S. health care system has distinctive features that allow it to be described as a kind of anachronism that miraculously survived to this day. Despite the highest medical technology, including technology of business governance and the best in the world scientific basis, the ideology of U.S. health care itself, in my opinion, is almost an exact copy of the system that was brought to America by early European colonists. Historians, if they wish, can recreate the average look of ideology of health care as it was in Europe in the middle of seventeenth and the beginning of eighteenth century, but adjusted to national identities. The only upgrade which the system has undergone during this time between patient and physician now appears as an intermediary: insurance company.

What are these distinguishing features? *First*, medicine remained relatively closed, a clannish profession, a type of medieval guild. Neither the state nor citizens until very recently were allowed into the 'guild kitchen', which adopted the technological and marketing solutions. The medical community there still stands apart from the rest of social institutions, largely retaining its medieval 'liberties'.

Second is the method of payment for medical services. The doctor gets education in a closed 'clannish' system for his money and then tries to justify the invested funds, providing services to citizens through business intermediaries, which are insurers and assisting companies. From the point of view of the doctor, his service is economically and fundamentally no different from repairing a TV or car in instalments. The social role of the state in such an ideology only recently attempted to wholly or partially participate in medical payments of citizens, and health care workers all in history made out a bill for their services, for both individual citizens and the state that paid for them. At the stage of the doctor's education or the stage of certification or the stage of practice and continuing education, the state does not claim its social interest in the results of the medical community as a whole, preferring to find out detours through educational programmes for potential and current patients and encouraging or fining certain types of businesses, including pharmaceutical, tobacco, alcohol, food companies, etc.

The *third* feature of the United States is that it continuously receives massive population from all the world, with the majority of the population having no experience of co-financing social insurance projects, or even if such experience is present, it is not compatible with different groups of immigrants. A large proportion of the foreign population leads to the fact that the United States still cannot create a complete system of health insurance for the entire population. For the state with such a structure of population, the risks of health insurance are too big and it is logical to put him into private hands, which by definition can afford to risk much more by artificially restricting the market and limiting itself to the most solvent parts of the population. This unique and permanent social 'instable routine' does not allow the U.S. health system become European, designated for 'stationary' population that is able to articulate their social goals and generate a social 'umbrella' of sufficient size to cover the majority of citizens. Such a health care system by their ideology is still a 'temporary' system that spontaneously arose in the era of the first settlers that are prone to constant changes of residence and is characterised by sharp social, material, and cultural inequalities.

There comes the understanding that this HCS, despite medical advances, as a separate service of a specific physician for a specific patient, starts to break down during the transition to fundamentally new technologies. The U.S. population has begun to notice that the price of such health care is prohibitive, and the accessibility of modern effective treatment is reduced. Medieval way of financing health care has become like a brake, in the sense that even the most advanced technology cannot show its effectiveness for society fully because of their low availability. The public opinion will begin to shift, aimed at greater social responsibility of medicine, at the fact that the population has begun to influence the clannish medical community, not so much in order to control 'what?' doctors make, but for the fact that people could make physicians also implement 'why?' and 'what for?' which in the immediate interests of doctors are not yet included. The book *Redefining Healthcare* by M. Porter and E. Teisberg is one of the attempts to indicate to the American (and not only!) society some oddities in the health care system that are becoming more visible to the professionals.

In this book in Chapter 8, 'Health Care Policy and Value-Based Competition. Implications for Government', the authors write:

> The fundamental flaw in U.S. health care policy is its lack of focus on patient value. (p. 323)

> If there is any overarching perspective that has guided public policy, it is government's version of zero-sum competition: drive down the cost of government programs by policing costs, forcing down prices, and shifting costs to the private sector. (p. 324)

> In all of these disparate views, however, there is agreement on one thing: the current system is not working. A fresh approach is clearly needed to address a

> health care system that is consuming a larger and larger
> share of public, corporate, and individual resources with
> questionable results. (p. 326)

Thus, the main words uttered are 'the current system is not working'! I think that it should be clear that a system that does not work could not survive a couple of hundred years, resisting any attempts to reform it. The point is that the system works, but for itself! There is no mechanism that would allow the system to produce the result, which it is expected. If it is more precise, nowadays the American society can begin to understand what exactly is expected from the system. I think that this is what the authors of this book are trying to convey to the reader.

First of all, it would be nice to understand exactly who competes with whom and for what resources? Porter says that medical providers compete for patients' money, and it's totally logical in a market economy, no more and no waiting. The means of competition are relevant in offering services that are the most appropriate to customers' expectations at a reasonable price. Porter says that this competition is counterproductive, because it offers a process, not outcome for the patient. It seems to me that the root of the problem is that the patient and medical provider traditionally understands by the proposed product that there are two different things:

- *Medical services provider* speaking about treatment refers to the chain of process steps, reaching the best possible results for some time and known money.
- The *patient* under treatment refers to the elimination of his medical and social problems to restore his ability to work within a certain time and fit in the available amount for him.

The only factors for which patient and medical provider can come together are the sum and time. If these conditions are met, the transaction is considered concluded. But the results of all medical procedures in general are probabilistic in nature, and the parties understand them differently. For medical providers, the result is a faithfully executed process chain, for the patient, there is restored workability or more years of life, and the first does not necessarily guarantee the second. All the many proposals of Porter in this chapter were reduced in order to force the medical provider to understand the results just as the current patient understands. But there is a huge problem: The patient obtains the explanation about the possible outcome from exactly the medical provider, i.e. someone who is financially interested in his misinformation to ensure maximum sales! Therefore, most of the conclusions of Porter in Chapter 8 focuses on how to organise the information field, which would be correct, impartial, and timely information for the patient about the best possible outcome for his medical condition.

I think that in reality the problem is even more complicated. There is competition among medical providers for patients' money—that's not all. In fact, all actors compete: medical providers, patients, medical insurers, and governments.

- Providers, as already mentioned, compete for money of patients and for now all the available potential patients, not just the population of this state. Limitation of this type of competition serves the cost of moving the patient from the residence to the provider of medical services. We should expect that as the solution of traffic problems and reduce the cost of moving people on the planet; the available pool of patients will increase and competition of this type will increase.

- Providers of medical services compete with each other also for the public funding they receive because of government's involvement in paying for medical services for some categories of patients and some socially important disease entities. The purpose of this competition may also get all sorts of preferences: tax, advertising and information, technological, political, personnel, and others, which allow access to new medical technologies and new pools of patients.

- In the countries that have HCS, which cannot evenly cover the entire territory of accessible medical service providers, patients compete for the possibility of getting even formal medical care. The advantages of such competition are awareness of patients about the availability of the medical provider, ability to quickly move around the country, and material prosperity, since under such conditions the prices will be unreasonably high.

- Patients compete for saving the maximum amount but achieve the desired result (not necessarily the provider from the current state). Under the 'desired result', they can assume quite different things, depending on the patient's understanding of his medical state and possibilities of modern medicine. In this competitive field, patients are divided into multiple pools with different requirements for the final results, depending on many factors: age, education, profession, awareness of its pathology, financial features (both personal finance and financial capabilities of their insurance company), etc. But subconsciously, all patients are well aware of finite resources of any health care system, and that fact encourages competition between them.

- Insurers compete, firstly, with each other for money of potential patients, and secondly, they compete with providers of medical services, by absorbing the money not only of current but also of future patients 'on the distant approaches' to hospitals and, thus, reduce the pool of customers who could pay providers directly for services. The fact that there is competition among medical services providers and the insurers for the finite resources of the patient, in my opinion, is insufficiently reflected in the literature.

- Insurers compete for the number of healthy population that is sufficiently solvent to pay for modern insurance services. The means to attract the customers to the insurer is the price and complete coverage of potential medical and social needs of patients. Limiters for such a competition are the laws of various states while the physical presence of the patient for the contract and the insurance payment is not necessary, and if it were not for these limitations, health insurers would have long operated on the internationalised pools of clients of enormous size; moreover, the contemporary banking services have already allowed that.

- Recently, insurers have begun to compete also for the opportunity to save on a denial of service to already sick clients or customers who often get sick. This type of competition arose after the state began to try and force insurers to work also with customers that are unfavourable. In fact, this is just turned out in the previous paragraph, but it should be recalled that it is an important motivator of behaviour of insurers in the market. To combat this phenomenon, Porter offers to 'create pools of patients at risk' and distribute them equally among insurers, thus making the market fairer in relation to insurers. However, to implement this idea, all insurers should be unified and equal in terms of prices and ranges of services provided, otherwise the situation will be unfair to customers. For now can only dreamed of this.

- The state competes with other states for the number and quality of current and future patients, for they are the taxpayers, working hands, and parents of future generations of citizens. Resource is the quality of life as well as duration of life that is offered to potential immigrants and their descendants. I want to emphasise that the state is the only player in the market that competes not for money patients, but for the patients themselves. Namely, the current and future patients are the basic value for it. Let's remember this fact.

That is to say, all of these types of competition in health care are aimed at making one or another way to attract and utilise the maximum amount of money of current or future patients. But funds that even the rich elderly citizens that often get sick of a given state can spend on their health and social needs are fairly limited. To broaden the base for competition and, thus, increase their income, market actors began to apply specific techniques:

- Customisation of health services, with medicines, serums, and medical devices (including implantable) developed specifically for a particular patient or a small group of patients. Price of the service while dramatically increasing, but the added value created for the customer is rather doubtful. But in the future, with the application of nanotechnologies, the customisation of medical services will become an integral and necessary part of making medical decisions and all medical activities.

- Compulsory insurance of the population dramatically increases the amount of funds available for consumption by competitors at the moment, but the problem is that the list of advanced technologies in medicine is clearly expanding faster than the list of medical conditions and methods of treatment that is covered by insurance. Thus, the probability that in certain circumstances and/or combination of diseases the patient will have to pay also for the newest treatment (that is not covered by insurance) is growing, which is the aim of competitors.

- There is active fundraising of patients from abroad, both as individual payers for medical services (now we call it medical tourism) and also as customers of transnational medical and social insurers and their alliances. State boundaries at this level of competition do not exist at all, and thus competition in the market of health and social services is no longer locked in their national quarters.
- International markets of semi-medical goods and services, including medical assistance, are developing. Special value to competitors represents technologies for lifelong support of a patient, while he cannot switch to another medical service provider for reasons of medical or technical nature.
- The use of telemedicine is a means to provide medical service to local or foreign patients without his physical presence, giving a sharp increase in the pool of potential patients which significantly save on travel costs. The market of telemedicine services currently shows one of the most impressive growth curves and promises to be a giant planetary market, as it is almost not influenced by local laws.
- Using the high availability of medical information to the end customer in the world today, health care providers purposefully create the fashion for certain medical technologies, causing inexplicable spikes of demand for scientists and developers and then cyclical disappointment in them though. Such information campaigns are a powerful way to create planetary demand for medical technologies' effectiveness which has yet to be proven and collect money patients *before* the publication of the late results of the given medical technology.

As mentioned in the previous sections, the only source of funds, consumption of which is the aim of the players on the medical services market and related markets, is the current and future patient which is now the whole world's population, while the citizens of more developed countries have more than the less developed ones. The population of economically developed countries is mere titbit simply because the average labour productivity in them is substantially higher, and respectively, the average per capita income is higher. That is, I want to say that for the money, for example, an American or Swedish pensioner now will indirectly fight simultaneously all medical providers in the world, as well as all providers of health and social insurance. The only player in the market, which will be interested not in the consumption of current and future patient's money, but in improving its quality with a reasonable increase in its quantity, will be the state. NGOs of patients, even global ones, will fight only for 'honest business', but no more for matters in general beyond their competence and interests. To expect from them requirements to better organise the HCS or to introduce advanced medical techniques to increase the number of people is as naive as to expect from the mall visitors the claims that the store has requested for additional buyers. The patient is a natural marketer; he knows exactly the fact that if other things being equal, the prices are as low as possible when there are fewer buyers; that's why the population is always sharply opposed to increasing its size at a rate at which this becomes evident.

Launched globalisation will lead to a more and larger percentage of patients being 'shared'. By analogy with physics, which recognises that all objects in the universe (even the ones that we can not detect) attract each other proportional to their masses and inversely proportional to the square of the distance between them, now we can say that the entire population of the Earth (and even part of it living far beyond civilisation) is indirectly included in the pool of holders of the planetary health system that has formed before our eyes and which tries to regulate the same planetary market of health and insurance services. As an analogy of the mass here, it is the financial ability of the client, but as an analogy of distance, it is the degree of his accessibility for the system. It remains to find out what will be analogous of inertia in such representations. I propose to announce the degree of loyalty a patient has for outdated medical technologies the analogy of inertia, while such a loyalty is a function of his age and degree of financial ability, i.e., to be approximately the same relationship as the inertia and mass in physics. The accessibility, I suggest, is the physical accessibility of the patient (without this it is hard to provide medical and social services) and the accessibility of patient's funds to use by the system.

As soon as competitors in the market of health and social services will go global, their competition will get new features, and, in particular, one can easily predict the following:

- Competitors will be interested to involve in the system more and more new customers; in the first place, the most affluent customers will be involved, regardless of their place of residence or citizenship. Thus, actors in this market will be indirectly interested in the fact that rich people will as much as numerous, and, in general, it is good.
- Competitors will seek to ensure that client's funds are in the form most convenient for consumption of the system, for which they will lobby for changes at the state level. Such changes may lead to a decrease in the degree of client control over the expenditure of his own funds and a view in which they are, and, in general, it is bad.
- The process of establishing global medical and social markets will likely try and undergo all the stages double quickly, which passed large-scale machine production in the early twentieth century, with transnational mega-corporations, attempts to monopolise markets, lockouts in the form of mass rejection of support of large groups of patients, strikes by patients in the form of a mass refusal to pay the bills, and other charms of a

little-regulated market. Any sudden movements at such a critical market for the population as the health care market is very bad, but for certain groups, it is even catastrophic. The only player at the outset who can lead a new emerging market in the civilised appearance will again be the state.

- Advertising on this new market will have features; as opposed to other goods and services, medical service can be tested by the client usually only once. Because the clients usually in such conditions cannot go to a competitor, competition tightens, respectively, and the pressure of advertising on its target audience will increase. The state here will need to intervene to protect the interests of clients in the early stages of market.

It is already seen that a difficult time is expected for the market of health and social services. In fact, it has already begun. Those countries that had begun to use new technologies not just of medicine but integrated chains of various medical and social technologies into one meaningful whole have abruptly pulled ahead in terms of providing additional value to their patients. What is the main additional value?

If you recall the birth of technologies of mass production of goods in the early Middle Ages, the main way to distinguish a quality product from an amateur forgery was the presence of trademark, which confirmed the qualifications of the master and his membership of the guild. Counterfeiting of trademark attracted severe punishment. Thus, the client no longer had to spend time for checking the quality of goods, but it was enough to see the trademark of a standard form. With the complexity of products, the ability of the client to personally evaluate the quality of goods fell, because for this, they needed to have sophisticated skills or create a special situation. How can you check the quality of the gun if you do not shoot out of it a few times? But what if you do not know how or cannot shoot? How can we determine the quality of a fabric, if we not wear it for many years? There is no other way to assess the quality of technologically sophisticated goods as entrusting it with its testing specialist. Thus, the responsibility for quality is automatically transferred from the individual master to the management of the relevant organisation that performs the quality control. What confirms the presence of trademark? It confirms that this master (or the whole team) produces consistently high-quality product. That master was able to get rid of the probabilistic results of the application technology of making this product, and its defects are minimal.

As described in the previous section, a university medical diploma at one time served as the trademark that allowed an even completely illiterate patient to easily distinguish a genuine doctor from the quack doctors, but it's still not a guarantee of quality service. The current state of the market of health and social services and, in particular, modern management techniques as well as quality control of services pretty much allow the probabilistic nature of medical services results to be overcome, while the patient obtains a new added value of enormous size—stable (option: guaranteed) quality of chain of medical services which ends with the best possible outcome. It means quality control in the form of new medical brands come to the fore in the battle for the customer. But the clients due to their incompetence are deprived of the slightest opportunity to personally evaluate the very complex multi-component medical services and look for 'trademark'. What namely does he look for now?

I think that a trademark now and in the foreseeable future will be performing the health systems of countries that were able to organise a continuous quality control of medical services in their territories. It is remarkable that this country does not necessarily have to be developed in the technological and purely medical sense. As always, when you go to a newly created market, competitors are on the same starting position, and past achievements hardly play a role. When Henry Ford applied the new principle of assembling cars, there was no technical innovation in this, but he was able to give the customer totally new quality and quantity of goods, which ultimately changed the whole country.

Thus, the name of the country turns into a trademark that guarantees the quality of medical and social services on the given territories. How long will it last? Probably not for long, because this technology is the so-called 'open source code', i.e. completely open to imitation. Dissemination of good management decisions in health care among states with political systems that will not prevent such borrowing will be held by historical standards immediately, and then only two brands will remain: a 'system with quality control' and 'system without quality control'. It is logical to expect that the new system will gain instant victory; that is, there will be no appreciable period of the struggle because the old system has no chance to keep the position, but it will not disappear completely, like the cottage industry didn't disappeared with the advent of robotic production lines. A man just likes to do something with their hands, showing his individual skills.

In the new system, the competition will take place already in the form of grinding of managerial techniques, in the struggle for a percent of successful results by reducing unproductive expenditures, for 'best design of medical services', that is, already semi-medical values, as well as in duration and ubiquity of 'warranty' of achieved results. Solitary handicraft medical providers remain to meet the needs of rare eccentrics who appreciate individual high art of the given physician at risk to get complications.

Next, in Chapter 5 in *Implications for Individual Physicians*, M. Porter and E. Teisberg wrote (p. 201):

- *'Medical practice must be designed around value for patients, not convenience for physicians.'* Apparently, the author here implies that the owners of medical institutions (federal government, state governments, local communities, religious structures, and private owners) need some organisational efforts to oppose the doctors (and medics at all) who are trying to get the greatest return and are creating businesses just for this. It is the peculiarity of the United States that all doctors (with rare exceptions) and much of the nurses are self-employed private entrepreneurs, the whole meaning of the activity of which consists of obtaining the highest possible income in the current legislation. For the implementation of this conclusion, the author would have them all as employees that would just change their system of incentives but at the same time, if I'm not mistaken, come into conflict with the letter and spirit of the U.S. Constitution, which provides freedom of entrepreneurial activity for all citizens.

I see only one way to realise the author's conclusion: deliberately pushing the patient and the doctor together in the same competitive field, namely, that the patient is able to demand and receive from the doctor the most value for his money—he must be a co-owner of medical structures and have a strong direct business mechanism to impact its functioning. The structure of the U.S. health care should be corporatised by patients, and one of the shareholders should be the state (governments at all levels), which also pursues its own, different from the patients, tasks of top-level management.

- *'The business of physicians is addressing medical conditions, not performing a specialty. Physicians must understand what different businesses they are in.'* Here, authors are trying to force the current physicians to become specialists in one or two diseases, but this situation the medical community is still considered a sign of low professionalism or even degradation. It's not so much a market problem as the problem of physicians' psychology. Centuries-old medical tradition involves a large element of universalism in this profession; a couple of hundred years ago, the concept of medical specialisation did not exist, yet the entire medical world was divided into surgeons and therapists. Now, M. Porter offers the next step in the specialisation of medical staff and its division into competing enclaves with various professional and business interests, which would automatically lead to the disappearance of the physician's profession, as we know it currently. The word 'doctor' will remain, but it will mean absolutely different. This has already happened in the past with the profession 'engineer'. Remember the universal engineer Cyrus Smith from the novel *Mysterious Island* by Jules Verne? And so these universal engineers are long gone, and in terms of contemporaries of Jules Verne, current engineers are not engineers; they are just professionals to develop extremely narrow classes of devices and structures. Market for design has matured and forced engineers to split into narrow specialties. Unlike doctors, engineers were not a clan with centuries-old professional traditions, and so, for them this division was painless. Specialisation of the medical staff in the patient's medical conditions is a very painful step for most doctors, but it's inevitable, and the authors are probably right. Customers with their money will force doctors to take the next step in their specialisation, not for this, but for the next generation of doctors. Just keep in mind that this specialisation is not the last; there is specialisation in the age of the patients, in their professional 'profile', on race and genotype, the geography of residence, type of environment and climate, and their combinations.

- *'Patient value comes from expertise, experience, and volume in particular medical conditions. Physicians must choose those medical conditions in which they will participate and achieve true excellence, rather than try to do a little of everything.'* I think the authors here are offering to split the proposal on market sectors before the splitting of demand happens. One can imagine a situation where a man in the late nineteenth century, wanting to buy a car, asks: 'Do you want sports car, SUV, or family coupe?' The client does not understand the question and says that he just wants to drive. In another situation, a customer comes into the store, just knowing that he needs a coffee mill. But at the entrance, he meets the manager who has a psychologist diploma. He stares into the customer's eyes and says that he, as a professional, believes that he needs a meat grinder. And the customer humbly agrees to pay for the meat grinder. Does this not remind you of our health care facilities? Before starting to compete for clients at the level of medical conditions, a doctor must undertake the set of measures, sometimes on the verge of detective investigation, in defining this medical condition. In such a situation, the narrow specialist is unproductive, especially if you have to differentiate a dozen fundamentally different medical conditions. Even now, in the presence of medical specialists universal in its field, the complex differential diagnosis often turns into a long process with nonzero probability of failure. How can the diagnostic process be built in the world where the doctors are divided and compete at the level of medical conditions, i.e. separate disease entities or its narrow groups? All of these specialists may take time in the diagnostic process as a sequential bypass, which is critical for timely assistance. Apparently, the diagnostics, as a form of medical practice, will have to be separated and excluded from the general field of competition, otherwise collusion between the narrow specialists and group that diagnoses medical conditions may happen. Do you remember the aforementioned manager that offered the meat grinder? Can anyone believe that he offered it unselfishly?

Another problem is the problem of full coverage of medical conditions. The fact is that they are clearly not equivalent in terms of complexity, time required for diagnosis, and treatment. In addition, they are very different in the effectiveness of therapeutic measures and the percentage of successful outcomes. What happens if the doctors in some area or the country will en masse specialise in the direction of the easiest medical conditions in terms of business? Who will do the treatment of labour-intensive and rare medical conditions? Who in such circumstances would impose on doctors the treatment of conditions that are unfavourable to them? Now such a covering happens because of the universality of physicians within their specialty; that is, after treating some unfavourable patient, the doctor immediately goes to the next favourable patient and makes up for lost profits. The imposition of such patients happens at the moment of splitting of the general medical field into narrow specialisations. If the doctors will determine the areas in which they are most effective on their own, it is almost guaranteed that all the areas that are uncomfortable for the treatment of medical conditions would be left out. Even if a doctor tries to specialise in such medical conditions, he will inevitably lose in the competition for the customer, because after developing the individual patients with this pathology in his area, he will be forced to become a nomad in search of casual patients. 'Shipping' patients to the narrow-specialised doctors will be several times more expensive than conventional wholesale delivery of goods to remote residence places—this is a feature of the market of health and social services, where not the goods are transported but namely the customers themselves.

- *'Health care value is maximised by an integrated team, not individuals acting and thinking as free agents. Physicians must know what team or teams they are part of, and ensure that these are functioning as teams.'* It seems to me that this phrase of the authors slightly exaggerates the situation. Certainly, service that is provided by a team will generally be fuller and better than the same provided by the single specialist. The question is: How it will affect the price of such services? Whether the entire cost of such integrated medical services will be approved by the patient as a thing he really needed and as exactly what he expected? The value of medical services for the patient is a complex set of factors such as quality of service, its price, the time needed for providing the service, his psychological comfort, waiting time, confidentiality, and much and much more. Do we not get the situation where by improving the quality of care we reduce other components of its value? I think that it will be better to stick to the principle of reasonable sufficiency.

Another problem is that narrow specialists belonging to different teams specialising in different medical conditions can and likely will compete with each other for the client because of the fact that they remain free agents in the market. The most valuable professionals become a bone of contention between the teams, which will lead to the fact that every team wants to have its own exclusive narrow specialist. The market of medical education will respond as it is accepted in the market: will start overproduction of narrow specialists compared with today; that is, if the number of doctors will be more, then their income will decrease. Thus, the application of such a principle can make the doctors oppose such changes.

- *'Physicians rarely have full control over the value delivered to patients, but are part of care cycles. They need to know what care cycles they are involved in, and how to integrate care with both upstream and downstream entities to ensure good patient results.'* The authors here, in my opinion, want to entrust the doctors with the role of system integrators who develop and maintain the 'interface' for a smooth and predictable interaction between professionals that make up the team and in between teams. I believe that the narrow specialist cannot be a system integrator in this case, as he will try to do administrative functions not intended for him, and even at the level at which he found himself. The more narrow specialist is the physician, the less he will be fit for the role of system integrator. This is a specific task of higher level management.

- *'Physicians have no right to provide care without demonstrating good results. Results should be made available to patients, other providers, and health plans as soon as measurement is reliable.'* Requiring is absolutely reasonable, but we will need to precisely define the words 'good results'; other health care workers may be subjected to targeted harassment, which is a type of competition under the banner of increasing value to the patient. First of all, we should understand they have to measure the results achieved by a physician or as a team relative to what or whom. Can we now compare the results of the example of Turkish and American cardio surgeons? Would it not be that after this Turkey would immediately close all cardiac clinics and stop all attempts to establish this type of specialised care? Is it fair to Turkish patients? Is it an acceptable comparison of the results of a specialised private cardiac clinic somewhere in New York City with the results of a small university clinic of the same profile somewhere in the outback USA? And how do we assess the value of such care for the health of the patients from the provinces, if it turns out that for this added value, they have to travel across the country to New York City and get it in a private clinic for a much higher price?

- *'Physician referrals should be based on excellent patient results, together with the ability of referred providers to share information and integrate care across the entities involved in the care cycle.'* Translating this requirement of the authors in ordinary language, we can say that the doctor should do analytical work to determine the degree of openness of the work of their colleagues (by what criteria?), the accuracy of this information (by what means and powers?), to build a registry of achievements (only now—on a global scale), knowing which care cycles his colleagues of other specialties are involved in and what is the degree of integration of his colleagues in these care cycles. Does it not seem to you that this activity, to say the least, is unusual for a doctor? From my perspective, this work is the power of a group of specialists, analysts, marketers, and system integrators, organised into a kind of national office with the prospect of transformation into a global organisation for the control of the quality of care. To require this from private practitioners, it means to try and discourage him from professional development, time for which does not remain.

- *'Electronic records and the ability to exchange and share information are indispensable to excellent medical practice. Physicians will limit effectiveness unless they wholeheartedly embrace IT.'* The question about the form of reports he sends to the doctors in regulatory agencies and to his colleagues is only a matter of speedy decision-making in the health care field. Exchange of information happens anyway and management decisions will be made anyway, but in today's world, it is critical, namely, the speed of the decision-making process. Avoiding the use of the fastest ways to share information is just as amazing as the attempts to control the country through the mails, which are carried in postal stagecoaches on the condition that you have a valid airmail and phone. The fact that many doctors do not use the electronic methods of information exchange is the result of the fact that in a professional environment there is no public demand for results in fast information integration of this environment because these results are not needed by doctors, so they do not increase their income and social status. This question is not for a doctor; it is a question to a state which does not expect (as opposed to patients) a significant improvement in the quality of medical services by introducing more rapid ways of information exchange.

- *'Physicians must seek out partnerships and relationships with excellent providers in their areas of practice in order to access knowledge and improve the integration of patient care.'* I believe this point is the most controversial. The main competitor of the modern doctor is his colleague, coinciding with specialisation and servicing the same pool of patients. Can you imagine the car corporation, which, referring to marketing research to improve the quality and after sales service of manufactured vehicles, suddenly began to build integration with other car corporations which were in the same market segment? And most importantly, will it open its technological developments for the greater integration for counterparts? Such processes in the business are called as mergers and acquisitions, and such things happen, as a rule, not voluntarily. In fact, the authors proposed to begin the process of creating corporations or medical cartels, which would virtually monopolise the local market of medical services for selected medical conditions. Firstly, such a practice is forbidden by antitrust law in many countries, and secondly, the first thing that happens after such a monopoly is the rapid rise in prices for treatment of above-mentioned medical conditions. The customer and his insurance company, as I indicated above, are practically deprived of the opportunity to try a particular medical service from different providers (as is observed in the production of ordinary goods and services); thus, they immediately become dependent on the producer of medical services closest to them, from which the customer will not be able to escape (as opposed to an insurance company that can change the provider). Thus, the only victims of such a market of medical conditions that is super-monopolised and artificially divided into small sectors will be patients.

Summing up, I agree with the basic provisions of M. Porter and E. Teisberg, where the general directions of changes in the future health care are shown correctly, in particular, the fact that the market of health and social services will be mature and divided into sectors within each medical specialty. The division will be based on medical conditions which are the most suitable for organisations of full cycle business processes with quality control to deal with the probabilistic nature of the medical service results. Following the segmentation of demand, segmentation of proposal will be logical; that is, the professional field of doctors and nurses in the next generation will begin to specialise in the treatment of medical conditions, a list of which will dictate the market. Next to this, the market of medical education will start to be segmented, which will produce much more narrow specialists than even today, but they will call them 'physicians' like before.

At the same time, the complex processes of extrusion of private insurers out of health care businesses and increasing the shifting of social insurance functions to the state and its subdivisions will take place. The state will more clearly show their social interest in the quality of health services and their cost and start with those medical conditions that are the first to come to the form of individual market segments with reliable quality control. After a while, the state will start to standardise the form in which current and future patients keep their funds in order to enable the health system to use them immediately, without lengthy procedures and delays. It is unlikely that this will be a special mega-community foundation; most likely it will be a new form of money, something like a virtual cash equivalent. Health insurance as a form of business in developed countries pretty quickly wanes, and this kind of competition will disappear in the near future. Market actors of health care and social services will more realistically envision the essence of the processes and predict the consequences of their activities in the medium and long term.

Patients for more effective control of the business chains and the quality of treatment will stimulate the processes of corporatisation of medical institutions and with the participation of the state force medical staff to implement a quality control system even for those medical conditions that are not quite suitable for this purpose in terms of medical business, achieving the highest coverage of the market and overcoming the resistance of conservative physicians with compensations and benefits. Patient in these circumstances will consider an attempt to treat him without quality control as an attempt to premeditated murder. States acting as the brands of health care systems will directly and openly compete with each other for complete coverage of medical conditions in the new quality control system, and the competition can lead to a kind of expansion; that is, more medically developed countries will provide assistance to people with certain medical conditions also not on its territory. In fact, this process has already begun. Providers of medical services will start to compete not so for the money of patients but more so for the mere fact of its existence in the system of quality control. Rare medical conditions and physicians who treat them will not fall into the new system; thus, they will be marginalised in the public consciousness of the next generation of patients, because they will look like artisans.

Managing the medical and social processes as a type of business with strict quality control and predictable results will be a very profitable service, as demanded by individual medical providers and entire states. We can predict an explosion of interest in new methods of quality control in medicine and marketing of health and social care services that are currently in the budding stage. At some stage, such management services will appear far more expensive than the actual treatment of medical conditions. Patients in the system in which the highest possible quality is guaranteed will compete for the opportunity to save their virtual money in choosing the right provider, which will offer the most comprehensive medical services for longer life of the customer and high quality of his life. At a certain stage of development of such a market, a new kind of competition for the new critical indicator will arise—extra years of life for patients and their more numerous progeny. There will be about this in the next chapter.

3. E. The New Patient and Macrohealth Care. Let's All Be Treated?

Just as macroeconomics considers the mass of buyers as the averaged agent in the market, calling it the word 'demand', which has the averaged needs, goals, and means to achieve them, it is useful to treat all patients as the averaged agents on the medical and social market, recognising that 'demand' in health care does not behave as a purely economic 'demand.' Thus, the new section *macrohealth care'* will appear in macroeconomics.

Also, just as macroeconomics describes the functioning principles of national and global economy, macrohealth care will describe the functioning principles of health systems in all aspects: social, medical, economic, medical genetic, demographic, legal, psychological, environmental, and others. The range of issues that fall in the consideration of such a science is huge:

- *Cycles in the national health care systems*: What is the growth of health care and why it is unstable? How should we determine the rate of growth in health care? What factors can affect the growth of health care? How does the growth of health care affect the development of the given country?
- *Ill-health*: Who are 'unhealthy'? Is ill-health either a positive or a detrimental factor for the economy and for health development in particular? How to deal with ill-health of the population? How can you identify the different levels of ill-health in the country? What does the ill-health affect?
- *The general level of prices in health care*: What is the 'general price level' in medical services market? How do the changes in the price level affect the health of customers? What is the inflation in health care? Which rate of inflation in health care is beneficial and which is harmful?
- *Money in Health Care*: What is the role of money in macrohealth care?

- *Budgeting of Health Care*: How does health care regulate its incomes and expenses? How do such criteria as welfare of society or the development of business in the country depend on changes in the health care budget, if any?
- *Balance in macrohealth care*: How does the country implement the international exchange of medical and social services to other countries? How do changes in exports and imports affect the cost of health and social services, the development of the given country, and the state of health care in the world in general?

Macroeconomics, if we use simplistic reasoning, explores the dynamic relationship between the changing needs of global demand on the one hand and the change in opportunities of global supply on the other hand and tries to meet those needs. All economic activities of people are always designed to meet their diverse needs. As the needs change into something significant, the economy will change as well. As mentioned, once health care is engaged it meets the most urgent, basic human needs that are inherent in biological species and cannot be changed, otherwise it will not be a human. Thus, it is permissible to say that macrohealth care is that section of macroeconomics which studies how to meet the basic needs of human, the ones that distinguish it from other species on the planet. I mean, that human needs include food and drink, sleep, safe housing, and a partner for procreation—they are common to all mammals on the planet and their satisfaction is engaged in the regular economy. But no animal on the planet other than the human can justify their need of having not just in offspring but healthy children, not just the need to preserve life but to have a healthy and productive life, not just in housing but in healthy housing . . . such 'strange' human needs engages macrohealth care. Unlike other animals, needs for health care services are the product of culture of this civilisation, and they can very quickly (by historical standards) change. Following them, the philosophy of the HCS is also changing rapidly The problem I see is that the legislative field of health care always more or less falls short of real needs of customers; one of the main reasons for this was described in the previous section, where the historical relationship of medical services and religious ceremonies was indicated. It is this constant backlog of medical and legal field is what customers perceive as a lack of health care system, as its inability to organise the service; in fact, this gap is just the inability of mass customers to insist on the accordance of the legal field and their real needs for medical services. Demand in macrohealth care represents the group of human needs that are most rapidly growing in size and changing by character, and according to the rate of changes, perhaps they can only be compared with the rate of changes in the IT market. Globalisation and rapid introduction of the vast masses of people of developing countries to the advanced culture makes the demand in macrohealth care one of the fastest growing planetary markets, which already have generally come into conflict with national laws. There are no chances for old laws to survive; it is already evident. This is as incredible as to expect that in order to save money humanity will cease to eat, sleep, or read the news.

In order to avoid catastrophic consequences in the form of the ubiquitous exit of health care practices from the legal field, followed by war 'all against all' in the unregulated global underworld market of health and social care products, there is an urgent need to see and formulate new demands of the old client or rather to understand why these requirements are changing and, most importantly, how they will change tomorrow. The proposal in macrohealth care should be *outrunning* instead of chronically lagging; moreover, it must participate itself in shaping the demand for services in the given field, just as it happens in other markets.

If we very briefly list the main changes in the social consciousness of modern health care, we can say the following:

- The sharp stratification of population in the sense of satisfaction of health services becomes apparent: The middle class can no longer meet their growing medical and social appetites, while the low-income class that is sharply growing as a result of migration to developed countries cannot meet even the simplest queries because the old funding system of HCS has not been designed for such a number of customers from the outset. In general, HCS of all developed countries have a large common drawback of their method of operation and funding; they almost do not take into account the migration of people and are not willing either to a sharp increase or a decrease in the population. Any deviation from the concept of 'static population' causes a panic reaction. The upper income level segment of the population of all countries continues to exist 'outside' the health care system because they do not use public funds and pay for medical services from their own account. This stratification is extremely annoying for most of the population of all countries, and this situation cannot continue for long.
- Most of the patients can see a huge gap in productivity between conventional markets and the global market of health and social services. They see a constant overproduction of goods and services in a normal economy and at the same time shortfalls in health and social services, expressed as a constant increase in prices in health care and increase in waiting lists for treatment in hospitals. They are inclined to explain in one way the deficiency of medical and social services: the reluctance of physicians to treat well because the increasing number of healthy people can reduce their income. Nobody can explain the true causes of physicians' low productivity, and that is very annoying to them.

- Practical needs of macrohealth care are not from case to case but constantly conflict with the national legislation of most developed countries. This is a permanent conflict in the field of transplantation of organs and tissues, the prohibition and permission of abortion and surrogate motherhood, cloning of animals and human, and trials of new drugs. Even a routine blood transfusion such as a transplantation of liquid tissue has met with fierce resistance among some religious groups, although all of mankind has long accepted the need and harmlessness of it on the basis of very long-term results (this technology is about a hundred years old). The migration of population for health reasons is increasing; that is, people have begun to choose a new host country because they have to perform complex or multi-stage medical services that they need, although it is banned in their country of origin. The population of the planet has begun to gather in groups, separated by their relation to the narrow medical problems that were not there some fifty years ago. And these groups will inevitably change the laws of the countries in which they gather to meet their needs.
- Patients are less inclined to pay for the treatment process and more for the results. A 'result', they understand, as stated above, is the decision of their medical and social problems fully and quickly, with certain guarantees of quality.
- The modern patient is less inclined to be satisfied with the quality of medical services which the closest medical provider offers to him. Travel expenses less and less affect the selection of the medical provider. The more developed is the country in the medical and technological sense, the less is the impact of distance on patient's selection.
- A modern patient for the most part is far more skilled when choosing a medical service provider than he would

do a generation ago. He now takes into account not only the price (economic) aspects but also the social aspects, time dimension, professional, legal, and other aspects of choice. The patient begins to predict their costs not only for treatment itself but also for costs for supporting the achieved results in the distant future.

- The concept of ill-health of the modern patient is many times wider than a hundred years ago, and this expansion continues. Past generations of patients would not even dream of seeing a doctor about those medical conditions about which they are visiting him now. From this point of view, the words 'citizen' and 'patient' may soon merge into the public consciousness; that is, all citizens will be treated as patients. Accordingly, the concept of 'healthy person' will change as well. I think this concept would mean a patient in whom currently no dangerous disease can be found that would affect his life or ability to work.

- In the minds of the modern patient, there is a huge gap between what he reads about the achievements of modern medicine or about the latest technological developments and the facts that he sees in the hospital nearest to him. Global information space and high-speed Internet play a cruel joke on him: He sincerely believes that everything invented in medicine should be immediately put into practice everywhere, even in very small and remote hospitals. In his mind, there is no place for information about the complex procedures for admission of new drugs and technologies into practice on the basis of long-term tests and procedures of evidence-based medicine. This is the big gap in the information policy of macrohealth care.

- Whereas before a citizen would rarely become a patient, and some citizens even never consulted a doctor because of initially good health or because of inaccessibility of health services for them, now more and more citizens of all developed countries spend most of their lives as a patient or a client of social support services. The population has become more and more accustomed to think and act as a patient, to feel itself as a regular customer of the health care system. In the twentieth century, every citizen of a developed country begins and ends his life in a medical institution, which is not yet a hundred years old.

- The average age of patients is increasing with all its consequences. Public consciousness of clients of HCS in developed countries is more and more similar to a nursing home client's consciousness; this is an entirely new problem, which greatly changes the face of the future HCS. Such a client for the most part does not want any new treatment methods and new medicines, does not like new people, and generally eschews any innovations. He tries to save money on that than dangerously save and then be happy to vote for the satisfaction of his folly. He is much more conservative and selfish than the younger patients. Budgeting of HCS under these conditions turn into an intricate task, especially when you consider that the management of such a system is in the hands of the same age group as the majority of elderly clients. I only hope that after a generation of old people in the mass, it will be different (see 1.F).

Summing up the section, one can say that the future doctors will be working much harder than today's generation. The future of health care looks like a collection of professional enclaves populated with highly specialised young physicians, who will spend most of their time not on patient treatment but on training for all new and new emerging technologies of diagnosis and treatment of narrow medical conditions, as well as legal ruses and subtleties that can protect them from penalties for treatment failure. Insurance for doctors and nurses from professional errors in these conditions can be a much more profitable business than the actual health insurance for patients. Medical legislation will disproportionately grow and begin to be segmented according to medical practice; there will be lawyers who will be specialised in transplantation law, pharmaceutical law, maternity, and even paediatric law.

The whole society will be presented as patients, including the embryos in the womb, since any deviation from the average-statistical indicators of health of any human being will be treated as a medical condition and as a subject for immediate treatment. Patients will be inclined to pay only for results achieved in the statistically average time terms. Dictates of the patients will also apply to medical methods used by physicians. Distribution of the latest medical information will happen with speed like news is distributed today in the world; therefore, a doctor who has not yet mastered a method of treatment that allowed one last week will be deemed to be not qualified. Improving the productivity of health workers will be a major challenge for all health care administrators because the flow of patients will be enormous, comparable to passenger transport flows for now. Patient care, including the proper medical and diagnostic activities and semi-medical business, will occupy an increasingly important place in the economies of all developed countries. The subject of 'macrohealth care' (it is possible that is under a different name) will be fairly common in the academic calendar of the leading universities and business schools around the world.

Medical enclaves at first will be grouped within certain states that according to the request of its people, would have adapted their legislation for specific medical procedures that are illegal in other states or questionable in terms of morality. Thus, the medical activity, better to say, medical tourism, will become an important component of national economies, just like some countries that are now largely living on tourism services. One can imagine a small and poor country that will change its law so that it can become a monopolist in the performance of any important medical services, implementation of which in other countries is associated with the legal obstacles and constraints. After a while, the country will not have to think about the development of its industry and agriculture, as almost all the clinics of that profile on the planet will now be created or will be transferred to the territory of the jurisdiction of that country. Highly specialised medical tourism could be a considerable source of income of this small country. Doctors of this specialisation will be proud to have the passport of that country, as well as lawyers specialising in this sector of medical legislation will be business agents of that country even if they do not want.

Medical monopoly will start to affect domestic and foreign policies of states; state officials will be involved in the alignment of business chains between countries, just as it's happening now between the different governments and multinational corporations. Such inter-state health care business processes will be the first steps in creating a planetary HCS, covering the entire population of the globe. WHO under these conditions will turn into a global marketing agency for the development of new medical services, the identification of new health and social needs of the ageing population, and the organisation of the training of medical staff for all new tasks. In the next section, we try to imagine how the average patient's life in such reality will look like.

3. F. Life As the Treatment Procedure

At the moment, every resident of any developed country becomes a client of its HCS immediately at birth. In recent decades in developed countries, there has been a steady trend towards increased medical surveillance for a new generation before birth, i.e. the embryo enters the system of such control at the time of diagnosis of pregnancy. Nobody is surprised now by the use of the phrase 'the diagnosis of pregnancy' as if it's a disease. For comparison, about 200 years ago, pregnancy of a she-patient during her treatment was absolutely not of interest to the doctor, because he had no practical means to affect the foetus and the course of pregnancy, but to break it in a completely barbaric way. Also, there was no understanding of how pregnancy could affect the course of various diseases and vice versa. In those days, the first contact with the newborn by a qualified physician only occurred during birth and only the wealthy clients who could afford to pay the obstetrician. Currently in the developed countries, all human embryos at the moment of their detection become objects of medical attention and, if necessary, the objects of prenatal diagnostic and treatment procedures.

The number of medical and diagnostic procedures performed in utero is growing; in this regard, sooner or later, the legal consequences will be sure to come, namely, the *recognition of the embryo as client*, although it may sound strange. Of course, such a customer would be legally incompetent, like a newborn baby, but actually it does not change—when a doctor provides medical services to pregnant, in fact, he has two organisms: the pregnant woman and the unborn child. Gradual recognition of the embryo and foetus as a subject of rights, including property rights, is inevitable. Because modern development of transplantation surgery will be particularly important issues of ownership to the organs and tissues, the question of the ownership of such a temporary organ of the human body like placenta also should be asked. In fact, to whom does it belong? The mother or the foetus?

Once the embryo and foetus become clients of HCS, it immediately changes the system of accounting and statistics in medicine as well. The fact that health care service is provided to the embryo will be reflected in the accounting system of medical procedures and health insurance, and even the financing of medical services. At the moment, the object of the financing of medical services is the mother, even in cases where the real object of their use is the body of the foetus, so now it is just much easier from financial and legal points of view. But in future, the foetus will have to be considered as a separate object of health insurance and, respectively, medical financing. The fact that the client of HCS is temporarily located inside the maternal body, which in turn is also a client of HCS, will not have any effect on the financial and legal issues.

Even the view of the population pyramid in the future may change. Now in the first lower line of the pyramid are children aged 0-1 year. Strictly speaking, this is not true, because these organisms existed nine months before, but just inside the organisms of their mothers. In HCS economic terms, they spend finances and other HCS resources for them, but they were written off by their mothers. It's perfectly logical to highlight these nine months in a separate bottom line of the population pyramid, which give more order in economic terms, but also clearly show for HCS officials that there is actually still a large part of the population in the country (about 1%), which is not visible yet, but you need to plan and spend resources for it (Fig. 3E.1). This additional line shown in the figure in black will a quarter narrower than the current one (nine months against twelve months of the first year of life) and a little longer for both sexes than the next, because, unfortunately, not all foetuses are successfully separated from their mothers' organisms.

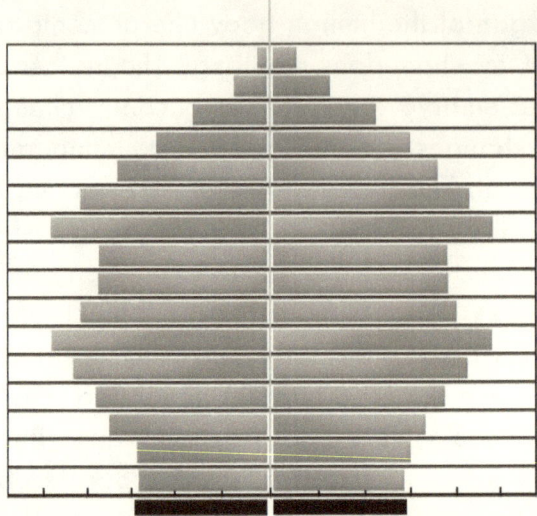

Fig. 3F.1. Proposed additional line of population pyramid (shown in black), which reflects the population which is not yet separated from the mother's body, but, nevertheless, consumes medical services and HCS resources. Explanation in the text.

Many of the issues that are now not even in mind are necessary to be decided for the future health care law professionals, in particular, the following:

- Issues of malpractice, when a medical professional provides unnecessary medical services to embryo, not knowing about his existence (providing medical services to pregnant woman before the diagnosis of pregnancy). There is also the question of the responsibility of the pregnant woman, who deliberately conceals the fact of her pregnancy from health care professionals that provide services.

- Issues of protection of the personality of embryo or foetus, as well as the state of his mind and the nervous system. As you know, a lot of food and drugs taken by a pregnant woman enter the blood of the foetus and change its state. The same applies to the strong emotions of the pregnant woman. The question for the future lawyers is whether the pregnant woman is responsible for the damaging effects on the mind and the nervous system of the foetus, which she could have prevented, but did not.

- When does an embryo or foetus begin to be the owner of organs that make up its body and membranes, as well as prosthetics installed into his body 'in utero'?
- Who is the administrator of these organs? Are these rights subject to transfer to other parties?
- Exactly who gives consent to medical procedures for embryo and foetus?
- There is a question of priority in the rescue of one foetus at the expense of another during multiple pregnancy, the legal responsibility for deliberately killing a foetus to save the life of another, and the differences of such a procedure from euthanasia.
- Will financial compensation for the harm caused by health professionals to the embryo or foetus be given in the provision of medical services and who is the recipient of the compensation?

Thus, recognition of the embryo and foetus as a client of HCS will change the relationships in the health and medical law and make lives of health care workers and pregnant women a little harder, but it will increase the degree of fairness in the delivery of health services and the degree of their targeting. It is possible that any future health services for women will begin with a pregnancy test, just to see what number of customers will obtain the service (one, two, or even three) and which actions will have to be performed at the time of service so as to not damage any of them. Future health professionals working with female patients all the time have to take into account the potential legal consequences of pregnancy and indirect provision of medical services to the client of HCS, which is inside another customer, and thus follow a complex system of priorities.

Based on the foregoing, medicalisation will cover all periods of the life of every member of society, including the prenatal period. This will expand the powers of health workers, but it will also increase the load on them, and without that, much responsibility already rests on them. It'll change the life of the foetus as well: Now from the detection of pregnancy up to separation of the foetus from the mother's body, he will be under the same supervision of the health and social workers as that after birth; thus, the fact of separation of the foetus from the mother becomes a private anatomical and physiological detail that will not affect the medical and legal status of the new member of society.

As soon as the *intermediate* medical technologies will be increasingly replaced by the *final* technologies (see 2.A), which will solve a specific medical problem for a given organism fundamentally, irreversibly, and forever, the intensity of medical procedures that occur in the in utero period will increase. From the medical, economic, and ethical point, it is advantageous to carry out all corrective and therapeutic interventions in the period before birth because in this period the adaptation reserves of the organism are the highest and the chances of getting complications are minimal. That is, the life of the foetus and newborn will be very active in the medical sense and will remind us of the finishing of products released at the factory as a typical variant, to adapt him to the given environment and the living conditions.

This kind of 'tuning' of foetuses and newborns will be very effective in economic terms, as they require much less resources of HCS in the future, after this generation reaches the age of workability. Microscopic doses of drugs for injecting, a very short healing time, the ability to produce even complex surgery in the outpatient department, the presence of the mother's body, which serves as a safety 'buffer' between the external environment and the patient inside and can be used as a depot of certain medications, as well as a dependable 'external' for foetus's circulatory and breathing systems—all this gives a huge advantage to perform all the unpleasant and traumatic procedures before birth. Purely technical disadvantages associated with the difficulty of access, the calculation of micro-dosage of injected agents, and miniature endoscopic instruments are solved by modern technologies. Thus, in the time before separation from the parent body, the newborn will be relieved of most of defects that are diagnosed by medical staff in the earliest stages of development. All of his medical conditions will be corrected or controlled; he will have a comprehensive medical 'profile', fully examined and ready for further medical support at all stages of his life.

In connection with the foregoing, many medical specialisations in the future can get their intrauterine (IU) versions; there will be new medical specialties, such as IU thoracic Surgery, IU neuro—and cardiac surgery, IU transplantation, IU endocrinology, and others. There may be even IU psychology and psychiatry.

As they grow older, the body of each child will be the subject of careful but unobtrusive monitoring of medical staff or, more precisely, of automatic recording systems, which if necessary will inform the responsible medical staff about the problem. In fact, modern technology already allows us to establish a continuous monitoring of the development of the organism; the question is only the price, which already pretty soon will allow their massive use. Diagnostic and measuring sensors can be installed at places of permanent residences of children (or covertly or openly in the form of toys or furniture) in preschools and schools, and they continuously measure and record the dynamics of many individual parameters, from simple height and weight to the frequency of breathing at rest and during exercise, body temperature on control points, pulse rate and some biochemical tests; for example, in the form of a game, you can easily measure the sugar content in blood and urine, make a picture of optic fundi, or measure the visual acuity and hearing of children. Such tracking technology for the development of children can largely replace clinical examination and most importantly take it to a whole different level of quality: automatic real-time analysis of incoming measurements, separation of young patients according to groups, on the basis of gender, age, social group, and the execution on the basis of these data the far-reaching conclusions for deficiencies in the education of children, their moving activity, and nutrition, as well as the identification of groups that require correction or treatment even before the problem is noticed by their parents or caregivers.

Maintaining such a system is actually much cheaper than clinical examination involving medical personnel for periodic medical examinations of all children and manual data analysis of the coming annual measurements and tests, like it was done twenty years ago. Manual input of results in database does not much help the cause, as it requires double work: Manual collection (reading) and manual data entry all of this work requires trained and highly paid personnel whose qualifications have be maintained between sessions of data collection. The use of such a system is in fully automating the process of reading, structuring, storage, and analysis of primary data with the exception of the human factor. Moreover, the frequency of reading data in this system has virtually no effect on the cost of maintaining a system, but it greatly affects the accuracy and timeliness of the data collected and, consequently, on the quality of the medical and administrative decisions. This system eliminates speculation, extrapolation and fraud and allows dealing only with facts. Humans involved only at the stage of the decision-making respond to the problem after initial data analysis.

Such a system would avoid unnecessary periodic medical examinations of children with screening tests; instead of this, with hidden accumulation and analysis of information, it will detect the narrow groups of risk in children and work only with them, providing a sharp decline, more precisely, the changing nature of the load on the paediatric service. Thus, children without exposure to pathology till a certain age will learn about the presence of medical staff in the society only from books and media resources and will not feel the fear of them, which will be very important for their unbiased attitude to doctors and health care system already there in adulthood. Also, children diagnosed with severe pathology that could not be completely eliminated during the prenatal period will receive treatment at as much as possible an early age, with a view to bring them to the end of the growth in the fully compensated form which is rarely possible now, because the basic resources of health system are spent on unproductive and time-consuming examinations, tests, and screenings for the child population of all age cohorts. Of course, saving resources of HCS on the growing generation is not an end in itself; the main goal of such forced savings is to have a head start resource for older generations, because namely they will be the largest and problematic customers of HCS in transition.

In Section 3.C, risks associated with the growing percentage of elderly population in developed countries were described; in that already in 2050, the percentage of elderly people may reach 40-45%. With such a shortage of workers, the only way for HCS is maximum automation of all that is possible and saving resources on younger cohorts. Active case detection and correction of children's medical conditions mainly in utero and in early childhood period is an effective way to save resources not only on the care of children but also on youth, because after such a treatment they will have a much higher initial level of health.

The main immediate challenge of HCS in all countries, but primarily developed, will be the problem of medical care for avalanche, the increasing number of old-aged and super-elderly (centenarians) clients. Some countries in anticipation of this is actively looking for ways to survive their systems of social and health protection; particularly in Japan, they are actively working to create robots to automate the care of the elderly citizens. In other countries, they will test a different method: try to attract the private business into this sector, artificially making it profitable by the concentration of older people in one place; in particular, many countries are planning to start building separate small towns for the old-aged with appropriate infrastructure, including medical, and have specifically created a private social service. Generally, the replacement of some government health and social services by trained and pre-licensed private agencies may be a cost-effective step in the transition period when the state will face local or global medical and social problems that may suddenly arise and need urgent solution in the absence of sufficient free funds and skilled government workers. That is, the task of the state in such circumstances may be reduced to setting adequate social and health aims and creating the conditions under which the solution of this problem may be interesting for specific businesses.

In the economy, which can already evaluate the effectiveness of their health and social efforts to identify and correct the medical conditions for any sex and age group, the design of therapeutic residential environments for groups with special medical and social needs can be effective. They may be resident populations for which the existing medical technologies were formally recognised as ineffective, and therefore, for the society it would be better to keep such people in special conditions under which they can live as long as possible and work relatively comfortable for them. Over time, some countries may begin to specialise in the creation and maintenance of comfort zones for specific population groups, especially since it may be associated with specific geological and climatic conditions, which can be a significant source of income for these countries or their separate administrative units.

Such scenarios of development medical and social technologies and international cooperation in this area may become a reality sooner than we think, because of the rapidly changing nature of production, which is less and less dependent on the physical concentration of workers in the place of production; as was for the industrial age, namely, the population became more and more free to choose the comfortable environment to live and work remotely. Such a comfortable environment can be both natural and artificial, especially adapted for living even for the small target groups. Even the fact of physical isolation (if necessary) of such a group can be fully compensated by its degree of integration into the information, industrial, and media life of the modern society as a whole.

As they grow older, if they wish the 'milestone-modernisation' technologies to upgrade their bodies can be used in droves, which will significantly affect the workability of these age cohorts in the future, the emergence of new (super-centenarians) cohorts, and change the course of action of future social services and financial burden on them in the developed countries, in particular, the following:

- Predicting the age of 'rejection' of the various organs and functional systems for different sex and age groups and producing pre-prosthesis (or the whole organ or its separate features), they can save considerable resources of medical and social services, freeing them for care in an emergency and unpredictable yet medical and social problem.
- Knowing the exact number of people who are carriers of certain medical conditions in each sex-age cohort in the future would give the opportunity to accurately plan the flow of medical and social resources and accumulate them in the appropriate places at the right time. In places of artificial concentration of carrier of certain medical conditions, they can create highly specialised social services (government, public, private) with much more degree of cost-effectiveness than currently.
- In cases of creating specialised residential areas for people with certain medical and social problems over time, they can create specialised health services, medical staff

of which are the carrier of the same medical conditions as their patients. In such cases, a greater degree of understanding the problems of the target group of patients may be achieved incomparably, with which there is a strong emotional bond, respectively, and a more targeted assistance, as well as more professional prognosis of the diseases and their complications.

- The ability to more accurately predict the appearance or decompensation of certain medical conditions in certain sex-age cohorts may provide the opportunity to accumulate individual resources of patients not 'in general', as is happening now with health insurance, but in a 'specialised' manner, creating target health insurance funds for certain medical conditions and for certain categories of the population, thus they will expend the funds in a much more targeted and efficient way, which essentially compensates the probabilistic nature of the onset of a particular disease in a particular age group.

- Funds accumulated by citizens in the form of individual insurance accounts for their non-use until a certain age when they may, with the consent of the owner, enter the total disposal of funds for the care of an older (previous) sex-age cohort; thus, better health of young population will automatically turn around a higher level of funding for medical services for older patients. Of course, these loans from one generation of patients to another one can only be made with a reliable guarantee that the next generation will also allow them to use their unspent medical funds.

- Housing environment in future may have gradations in terms of risk of onset of certain medical conditions for population living constantly in them. This refers to the level of potential trauma in this environment, the risk of cardio-vascular problems, the probability of poisoning or the accumulation of certain toxins, the probability of infection by certain flora, the likelihood of certain diseases of the skin, the likelihood of cancer pathology, likelihood of causing harm to the unborn on longer stay, etc. Current technology can express such probabilities in numbers and link them to the terms of permanent residence in that environment. These gradations of danger for the population as a whole and for individual sex-age cohorts can be used to calculate the correction factors by which the insurance funds or companies specialised in certain medical conditions can share resources, concentrating them in places where the pathology may most likely be.

In such circumstances, the person's life is gradually transformed into a *continuous medical procedure*, which may not be seen by patients, and the treatment and correction will be implemented not only for already diagnosed medical conditions but also for those that with a very high degree of probability occur in a latent state, but these cannot be accurately diagnosed by the current degree of sensitivity of diagnostic equipment and sometimes even for those that with a high probability will develop in the near future for the given sex-age group of the population. In the future, doctors will have to answer strange questions about their patients, such as the following: 'The girl out of eighteen years lived for five years in city "A". Before that, she lived for thirteen years in city "B". Her parents had lived for twenty-three years before she was born in the city "C". The question is what medical conditions related to living in these areas, with the highest degree of probability, will evolve in the next five years? What resources should be prepared by HCS in the residence of the patient for her treatment or medical correction?' The ability to answer these questions is the condition for the survival of the future health system.

Summary of the Third Chapter

So in the third chapter it was suggested that the health system in the near future cannot survive without coming to a new level and will not put themselves new, more general purposes. Moreover, it will have to include a new meaning, which previously either did not exist or was called by another name and was considered as a separate entity.

First of all, humanity will have to do the *humanistic* goal-setting in health care, after the qualification of this concept. Apparently, such a clarification in the future will have to do quite often with the development of society. Social guarantees of the state, which in developed countries now tend to sound like '*I'll compensate your expenses to overcome any medical and social problem, provided that you are a citizen of this state,*', will be translated into the biological plane, meaning that all those belonging to the species Homo sapiens will be subject to the guarantees of health and social care at the current level of technology, but the questions of the adequacy of resources will be taken away in the background. Thus, HCS will tend to *biological* warranty of care.

It was further stated that the future health care system will be managed in a fundamentally different way. As soon as the modern society will increasingly take on the traits of the global Internet community, HCS will have to be transformed in the same direction. It will have to be managed as an online community of patients, who will be all of members of the community by definition. A significant part of management tasks at the grassroots level will have to be delegated to the patients as well as to their cumulative processing power, which will produce a preliminary analysis of the collected data. This approach will help to get away from the control of processes and start to *manage the results*, not only in the narrow-medical sense but also in the social sense. The peculiarity of such a management is that problems at all levels (end phase points of development) need to be posed in the clear.

In such circumstances, a professional manager in the health sector is the person who directly determines the image of the future population, its physical and psycho-emotional profile.

Furthermore, it was noted that the growing demographic problems in developed countries very quickly become common, i.e. inherent in all countries and regions in the world, which will completely change the method of funding of planetary health care and will force it to automate the functionality, especially the management at the grassroots level. It has been suggested that the society will soon face a severe shortage of workers in general, and social and health care workers in particular. In 1950, the elderly in developed countries was about 5%, while in 2050 there will be about 40%; that is, there will be an eightfold increase in just 100 years when essentially the same medical technologies and the same way of social care will be followed. After a couple of decades (in 2070), the situation will become even worse, as even smaller and smaller age groups will become workable.

It was said that for the society in the demographic transition, the presence of modern health care system is a *matter of physical survival in general*. It was also stated that the changes in reproductive behaviour, which quickly spread to all countries, happened also due to the changes in philosophy of development and actions of the modern HCS. Apparently, in future, the migration processes will affect the structure of the society almost more than the mortality and fertility.

The market for health and social services will be more mature and will be divided into sectors within each medical specialty. The basis of this division are medical conditions; the most suitable for the organisation around them are the business processes of a full cycle with a quality system to deal with the probabilistic nature of the results of these services. At a certain stage of development of such a market, there will a new kind of competition for a critical indicator—*extra years of life of the patient* and his more numerous offspring.

The emergence of the section *macrohealth care* in macroeconomics was predicted. Macrohealth care will describe the functioning principles of health systems in all aspects: social, medical, economic, medical genetic, demographic, legal, psychological, environmental, and others. It has been postulated that macrohealth care should be outrunning instead of chronically lagging; moreover, it must itself participate in shaping the demand for services in the given field, just as it happens in other markets.

In the future, a person's life is gradually transformed into a *continuous medical procedure*, which may not be seen in patients, and the treatment and correction will be implemented not only for the already diagnosed medical conditions but also for those which occur with a very high degree of probability in a latent state, but they cannot be accurately diagnosed by the current degree of sensitivity of diagnostic equipment, and sometimes even for those that will develop in the near future with a high probability for the given sex-age group of the population.

Chapter 4

Scenarios of Medical Technology till 2050

After reviewing the causes of birth and evolution of the existing HCS in the preceding chapters and outlining in general terms the contours of the future HCS, it would be logical to move and attempt to delineate how future medical technologies and their combinations will change the philosophy of health care and vice versa and how the new philosophy of HCS and social services will require the development of specific medical technologies. In this chapter, I will try to do a very ungrateful thing—predict the overall scenario for the next forty years, i.e. the lifetime of the present generation of physicians.

First of all, is there a practical sense in being such forward-looking? And anyway, why should we try to predict events?

4. A. What Is the Point of all These Predictions?

All attempts to detail the shape of the future somehow a posteriori look ridiculous, if not pathetic.

(Boris Strugatsky, 1933-2012)

Futurologists have long noted that the larger the scale of the proposed changes, the easier and more accurate it is and the longer the time that they can be predicted. The larger the process than smaller random processes involved in it, the lesser the impact of these separate processes on the common picture and the finer patterns become visible, according to which the numerical characteristics of a more general process change. Of course, the more the short-term forecasts are required, the more accurately they can be made on the basis of the investigated trends of the present and the past.

But what do we mean when we talk about the *future*? The future exists in the human mind always in several layers and always has been. This is especially evident when we study foreign languages—it becomes visible that in languages there are always several instances of future tense, for that matter, as well as past tenses. In our own language, we do not notice it. These future tenses are formed, depending on their distance in time and whether they're perfect, that is, whether they are still in the process of the occurrence or they have already taken place? What is the 'future' in the everyday sense of the word? Any mention of the events of the future carries a prediction, in a sense, guessing. Predicting the future in a very short period of time for the average person has little value and, strictly speaking, is not the future. In fact, who can be interested in what will happen in ten minutes on the next street, but for certain narrow occupational groups (e.g., fire, police, or military in the hot spot), this prediction can be critical. On the other hand, the prognosis of very distant events (such as events which can occur after 20,000 years or more) for a person is not critical and does not cause any particular emotions, because he knows that this forecast will not affect his own life or the lives of his direct descendants. Thus, the person is most interested in quite a specific period of the future: the remaining years of his own life plus the lifespans of his children and grandchildren; in total, it will be 150-200 years. It is this period we call for now 'future' in the everyday sense of the word.

It is logical to assume that with the increase in the average life expectancy (ALE) in developed countries the concept of the future will change, and it is changing. If you say, at the beginning of the twentieth century, life expectancy in the developed countries was about 50 years, then we can calculate which period was then considered as the future for the twenty-year-old man: 30 years (his remaining years) + 40 years (the time at which his grandchildren survive him) = total of 70 years. Currently, in the developed countries, ALE is approaching eighty years, however, and the average age of childbearing has increased and is not on the level of 20 years, as it was in the beginning of the twentieth century. That is, for now the calculation of the concept of future for the twenty-year-old man might look like this (assuming that the age at first birth is twenty-five years): 60 years (his remaining years) + 50 years (the year in which his grandchildren survive him) = total of 110 years. Future has significantly lengthened, by more than a third. In fact, such calculations are not correct more, because now we cannot know how much on average our grandchildren will live. Mankind has entered a period of almost vertical growth of ALE, so our grandchildren can live many times longer than our generation. Thus, the term 'future' now becomes unpredictably longer. We are beginning to wonder what will happen after 200 or even 400 years.

But why do people want to know the future?

- It is well known that man is *curious* by nature. The more closed some information or area of knowledge, the more it evokes curiosity. People used to assess the social significance of themselves and others by the number of classified information, which that person owns. The champion on the degree of secrecy is the information about the future; people who claimed that they knew at least some evidence of the future have always enjoyed and now are widely respected and even the objects of mystical worship.

- People want to *prepare for the near future*, especially adverse future, so as to have the advantages compared with improvident and incurious neighbours. That is, knowledge of the most probable future is a factor of intraspecific competition in humans. A person wishes to convey knowledge of the more distant future to their offspring as well, making them thus more ready for it and increasing their chances of survival.

- The person makes predictions *for correcting his actions* that are based on it. Such predictions can drastically affect the choice of profession, choice of country of residence, the choice of the control of given country and its legislative field, the behaviour strategy, and the planning family. Thus, the projections, even those not quite scientific, affect life today.

- Man makes predictions for *learning how to do them*. Forecasting the future of varying degrees of remoteness in its various aspects is classical analytical task, for which there is a developed set of techniques, from the completely absurd to those quite serious, with the use of mathematical modelling and the whole modern computing power. Sequentially comparing issued forecasts with actual future, analysts sift through inefficient methods, thus turning the prediction of intellectual trick to real science.

However, forecasting of calculated events and forecasting trends and scenarios in the certain fields are quite different things.

In the first case, it is just a matter of proper plotting one or more mathematical functions, one of the coordinate of which is time scale (a typical example is a short-term weather forecast); in the second case, we have to deal with the resultant of a large number of countervailing processes that are fundamentally different in nature and are interacting at different levels. Besides them, there are also mutual influence processes, the nature of which is not yet understood. The only common coordinate for them is the same time scale. A special challenge is the fact that their time of interaction is a random variable.

The scenario of development in certain areas of human activity, in fact, is a sequence of changes in applicable technology, including also the technology of thinking, which is also gradually changing. Any long-term change in human needs, sooner or later, brings to life a new technology. An interesting question is: why does not every discovery or invention become the new technological breakthrough? Why new discoveries are often 'out of time' and what does it depend on? What is needed to discover something on time, just when it's needed to create a critical technology?

It is well known that the *Hero of Alexandria*, the great ancient mathematician and engineer, in the first century of our era had created a toy-turbine. He called it *Aeolipile*; it represented the first steam turbine—the ball rotating with the force of jets of steam. Why did not he go further and create a true steam engine? Was there no need in it? Did ancient people not need a powerful engine? Further, it is known that in China that gunpowder has been known since ancient times (at least since the tenth century) and was used in fireworks and mines. Why the Chinese have not taken the next step and created a true firearm? Unlike all the rest, humanity needs the new effective weapons forever. What is the problem? Why do people often not notice the new technologies, even when there is a hand just in reach for them? I think that the problem on closer examination is divided into several parts.

The *first* is that the requirement of satisfaction, which will use the new technology, should really exist in the public consciousness, and awareness of the need should occur before a discovery or invention. Not only should the inventor be needing this technology, but, namely, the large part of society should feel the need for it. Humanity must 'wait' for this technology. Returning to *Hero* and his contemporaries, it should be recognised that in those days there was no true need of the engine; we only ascribe to ancient people such a need from the position of the present day. The horse traction for those tasks the people set for themselves was enough. They just did not set the tasks that went beyond technologies they knew. Why is another matter. In particular, from time immemorial, mankind has dreamed about bird flight, but despite the fact that in ancient times it had all the materials to create a primitive hang glider or paraglider, they were not created because the human stubbornly wanted to play back, namely, flapping bird flight that is physiologically impossible for a human.

Second is that the practical application of the invention should not require new discoveries and inventions; that is, it should be possible to implement it right now. Mankind, until recently, was not able to store inventions 'in reserve'; he acted in his collective behaviour quite like ancient hominids, just throwing a strange item found on the ground and continuing the search in the area of the already known, which the mankind knew and was able to apply. Stories how people 'remembered' previous inventions and used them later when they realised that it was discovered are rare and painstakingly assembled in the school textbooks, precisely because they are so rare. Also, the time that has elapsed since such a discovery is usually small and does not exceed the lifetime of one generation. The memory about inventions that were done, but not those that were used, was not passed down to descendants because such knowledge in our brains was considered useless. All cases of 'selection' of previously done scientific discoveries and inventions have occurred at a time when it already was the practice of scientific publications, albeit negligible circulation. Namely, the possibility to collect publications about 'strange facts' and discoveries enabled humanity to dramatically increase the effectiveness of scientific research and the speed of the creation of new technologies. It can be said that the present system of scientific publications is the 'operational memory' of humanity, whose main work is on the creation and understanding of technologies.

Third is that the move to the new technology should be ready; the scientific base, in particular, should be a ready tool for monitoring and measuring the results of the new technologies. Mankind understandably avoids the use of technology, the results of which cannot be measured and predicted. This is especially true of medical technology. What prevented, for example, the great Galen from performing surgery on the internal organs, because all that was needed (steel tools, silk thread) already may have been manufactured? Why did these curative technologies not appear in ancient times? Apart from religious prejudice and lack of pilot experience, I think the reason is also the fact that at that time there was no social demand for such a treatment. There can be no effective technology for the treatment of diseases that are not yet known and the symptoms have not yet been described. But the methods of treatment of fictional diseases have always existed. If a modern surgeon were to be in ancient times and would have tried to apply his skills by diagnosing the modern medical conditions and performing the complex surgery, it seems to me that he would not achieve recognition and success in such a society. No one would simply understand what he did and what he treated. And most importantly, anybody would not call such an activity as treatment, because they would not have the tools with which at the time one could assess the improvement in health outcomes after these advanced treatment techniques. In other words, for starting the use of a new technology by mankind (even if invented accidentally or borrowed from someone), it should be able to detect and accurately measure the effects (positive and negative) which were produced with the given technology.

Thus, the emergence of breakthrough technologies in medicine and public health can be expected:

- A problem which the new expected technology may solve will be recognised by the majority of the population in developed countries, not just by scientists working in this narrow field. *Forecasting of solutions of medical problem, even not entirely of scientific methods, produce a wave of interest in it among the general public, thus increasing the readiness of the population to solve it and shortening the period of adaptation to the new reality.* The more the public is ready to solve the medical problem, the faster is the true clinical decision, simply because they will direct much more scientists and material resources (public and private) at finding a solution to a given problem;

- The desired effects of the use of this technology will be clearly defined and the specific tools to monitor the results of its application developed. *Forecasting allows clearer understanding: firstly, what is the solution we want, and secondly to see which solutions we do not want, and to prepare in advance all techniques to distinguish the first from the second.*

- All the related technologies, including management, materials, personnel, human psychology, law, mathematical tools, and computer resources, are prepared in advance. This is one of the longest stages of preparation for the transition to the new technology. *Prediction gives a tremendous head start to create the entire infrastructure, allowing instant and widespread move to the new technology as soon as it will be discovered, receiving a maximum effect and minimal complications.*

4. B. Bionic Prosthetics. Copyright on the Structure of Human Body?

Mankind from time immemorial has dreamed about organs that other animals have, but that might be useful to man in certain situations. Entire religious and mystical cults gave rise to imaginary owners of super complete organs in different nations around: people with 'wings like an eagle', 'claws like a lion', 'eyes like a cat', 'legs like an antelope', and 'gills and scales like a fish'. Man that lived in a natural environment almost always had a sense of deprivation; he could not boast about organs, which would give him a decided advantage over natural predators or potential prey while hunting. He could not compete with any animal-specialist, neither in speed races with antelope, nor in power with a lion or a bear, nor in night vision with the cat, nor in endurance with the buffalo, nor in speed with an attacking snake, etc. After moving to the artificial living environment—the cities, people stopped dreaming about additional animal organs; in the city they were useless. And just after dropping out of the competition with the wild animals, people realised that the organ that could give them a decisive advantage over wild nature was always with them and worked fine all the time; this was their brain. Thanks to it, a man was sure that he did not need to compete at all with wild animals.

However, already in ancient times, there was a tendency to understand that the people are still in need of some improvement in their bodies. Increased life expectancy has led to the fact that middle class people massively survive diseases that used to be a rarity. Also, some age-related failures of organs were added. The time of the productive life lengthened so much that there was an urgent economic need for an extended 'shelf life' of the most wearing down of human organs. Added to this, there were the effects of injuries received in the fighting, because large and small wars were fought almost continuously. Already in third to fourth centuries BC dentures were first made, which were to replace the removed or fallen teeth. Artificial incisors carved out of ivory were implanted in rich Phoenicians, who fastened these prostheses in the mouth with a gold wire. In the Middle Ages, pig, dog, and sometimes human teeth were used as prostheses.

Primitive prosthetics made instead of lost limbs were known from very ancient times and in different nations. Hardly anyone would claim to know the date of manufacture of the first prosthetic limbs, especially as they were often made out of the most available material—wood, and therefore, only ones with metal parts have survived. Two thousand years ago, the Greek historian Herodotus told about a warrior who cut off his own chained foot to escape from captivity and many years later walked with a wooden leg. During the excavations of the Italian city of Capua, archaeologists found a bronze leg of a Roman legionnaire who replaced the leg lost then in a battle more than 1,500 years ago. In the Middle Ages, the artificial limbs began to become mobile. Certain prosthesis parts were connected with hinges as 'joints' and set in motion by the muscles of healthy parts of the body through an intricate system of levers and band traction. Prosthetic of ears and noses that were used by wealthy people sick with leprosy were also popular, which was then a scourge of big cities. With the technology of processing of coloured glass, the prosthetic eyeball appeared; it is of high quality, even by today's times. In 1249, the drop in cooled glass attracted the attention of a glassblower. The master picked it up and saw that he was able to increase the objects, and then he had the idea to use this feature for the correction of senile vision. Thus, it was the first documented prototype of glasses. Roger Bacon wrote about the use of glasses with convex lenses for the treatment of hyperopia for the first time. The high cost of lenses made them available only to the wealthy. But even the rare and expensive glasses made the productive age of people in intellectual professions much longer, which immediately affected the quantity and quality of information transmitted to the next generations.

As soon as the life expectancy in developed countries increased, the need for prosthetic organs that were refused due to age and their individual functions grew. The role of the prosthesis was initially purely cosmetic; they imitated, sometimes very roughly, the presence of the lost organ. To speak about the full workability while using the prosthesis is impossible. The only prosthetic functioning organ that really enhanced the workability were the same glasses, though they were used by a very thin layer of the population: the elderly wealthy intellectual professions and individual masters working with small objects (jewellers, watchmakers). Almost simultaneously with glasses, the prosthetic outer ear appeared: auditory tubes, whose role was limited to the direction of the sound waves as close to the eardrum of the deaf person. The most successful and one of the most ancient devices was the lost leg prosthesis with a sleeve that fit over the stump and restored the support function of the limb quite well at that time. As technology improved, the spectrum of organs and their functions that are subject of prosthetics steadily grew. There was for now a social component of prosthetics; it was no longer a private matter for the patient, but also the social task, giving such a patient an opportunity to socialise and allowed the society to save a considerable amount of funds that would have gone into the care and pension benefits for these patients throughout the country. Prostheses have been used namely for workability rehabilitation of certain categories of patients. They began to use prostheses immersed in the patient's body—the idea is not new, but it has received a new breath with the creation of new materials that can withstand the chemically aggressive environment of the body. In the past, the inner prostheses were only the gold and silver plates (later—steel) for closing skull defects after trepanation.

Prosthetics has become an important area of contemporary social and medical technologies to solve many problems:

- Socialise the patients with certain disorders that earlier had simply dropped out of society.

- Save the workability of patients, which would have a significant economic impact on a national scale.
- Give these patients the possibility of family life, participation in the upbringing of children and grandchildren, participation in education of the next generation.
- Develop technological approaches to the next level: the complete replacement of some organs of the body, expanding the range of their functions and then creating the fundamentally new organs that people would require under certain circumstances, due some of the professional needs or in the special living environments.
- At some level, prosthetics can be used to improve the communication capabilities of initially healthy people, creating new ways of socialisation of the population, the acquisition of new work skills, and the emergence of fundamentally new jobs and new careers.
- Prosthetics can completely change the face of preventive medicine in the near future; in particular, it may be possible to change the properties of human organs and systems so that age-related failures do not occur at all or occur at a much later age. It may also be possible to protect some organs and their functions in advance from injuries and damage in some particular profession or in some age groups.

As soon as human began to more deeply study his own body on the micro level, as well as other living organisms, he began to notice that many of the technological solutions for which the mankind had spent decades had 'invented' nature a long time ago and successfully functioned in terrestrial organisms. Moreover, people still cannot replicate some natural discoveries and inventions with today's technology. In the late 1950s of the twentieth century a new science appeared—*bionics*.

Bionics (also known as biomimicry, biomimetics, bio-inspiration, biognosis, and close to bionical creativity engineering) is the application of biological methods and systems found in nature to the study and design of engineering systems and modern technology. (from Wikipedia: http://en.wikipedia.org)

Differences: *biological* bionics studies the processes occurring in biological systems, *theoretical* bionics builds the mathematical models of these processes, and *technical* bionics applies the theoretical models to solve engineering problems. That is, all science actually consists of the fact that researchers are trying to borrow the solutions from the nature, using the fact that they are not protected by patents. Most of the natural solutions cannot yet even 'read', and those that have been able to understand cannot always be applied, since this requires very special materials.

I think that in the near future bionics will go through another qualitative leap—the transition from copying the natural solutions to the construction of biological objects with specified properties. This will have to solve several major problems:

- Create a group of materials which are fully biocompatible. As a first step to solving this problem, materials should be used that are compatible with certain tissues of the human body.
- Create biocompatible materials, which could respond to changing conditions, at least by 1-2 parameters and at least in the narrow range of changes.
- A separate task is to decipher the code by which the nervous system controls the peripheral organs and, above all, the organs of movement. Artificial neuromuscular synapse will be a breakthrough invention in this field.
- Creating a set of materials that to realise their functions could use (firstly—at least partially) the energy that is stored

in chemical form in the body. Creating a biomaterial, which would be manageable shortening in response to a nerve impulse (artificial muscles), is in my opinion the most urgent problem.

- Create a complex of biomaterials that can synthesise some given simple molecules from raw materials available in the body fluids, consuming the energy supplied by the body in the chemical and thermal form (artificial gland).

The first step in the development of new opportunities is coping with the already known solutions; people always start with this. In the first step, organs with low intensity of metabolism and that have rigid shape due to a significant mineral content (i.e. non-living materials) will be used. The first such organ is bone. Creation of an artificial bone or at least technology that allows bone to grow into the living matrix while maintaining its original form will be the breakthrough in the treatment of the majority of bone diseases, as well as injuries of the musculoskeletal system. Bone if broken or struck by the pathological process may be immediately replaced with an artificial one, not wasting time, resources, and effort on the extremely long patient's treatment. In addition, this technology will dramatically (at times) reduce disability from injuries and bone tumours. After some time, it will allow to create new, super complete bones to solve various problems, mainly the biomechanical.

As soon as a mass of various achievements of bionics will be introduced in the patient's body, and all these achievements will have specific authors and the patents the specific owners, a question will appear: At what point, the patient will be the subject of patent law and, accordingly, the patent protection?

As known, the subject of patent law is as follows:

Invention: *'As an invention protected a technical solution in any area relating to the product (e.g. device, substance, microorganism strain, cells of plants or animals) or process (process of affecting a material object with material resources). Invention shall be granted legal protection if it is new, involves an inventive step and is industrially applicable'* (Wikipedia). If the 'impure' solution (invention) from the patent point of view was used as a means of treating and/or prostheses, penalties were imposed on the beneficiary of such a solution. After all, beneficiary of this operation is also the patient himself. How to resolve the conflict, the more so because, as a rule, it will be impossible to extract such an invention from the patient? In other words, would the patient pay not only to the surgeon and to the manufacturer of implantable devices but also the owner of the patent for this devices?

Utility model: *'As a utility model protected the technical solution relating to a device. Conditions for patentability of utility model will be the novelty and industrial applicability. The legislator does not require inventive step for utility models. As can be seen from the definition, as a useful model can be recognized technical solution relating only to the device, as opposed to inventions which, in addition to the device, may be a substance, a strain of microorganisms, cells of plants or animals, the process of affecting a material object with material means'* (Wikipedia). Let's say that a patient used the treatment/replacement, which is not an invention but has novelty and wide applicability. What would happen if the term 'device' will be transferred on all the patient's body? After all, you can easily imagine the prosthesis, which is not possible clearly to localise in the body of the patient (the simplest example—artificial blood or pool of nanodevices enters in the patient's blood). Future lawyers may have to deal with the object of patent protection, which has the surname, passport, and own opinion about what is happening!

Sample of industrial design: '*As an industrial design is protected the art solution of the issue of industrial or handicraft production, determining its appearance. An industrial design is very different from the invention or utility model, it even looks like one of the objects of copyright, as it has in conjunction with the artistic design also the constructive solution*' (Wikipedia). Many of the solutions in the field of reconstructive surgery and prosthetics also have aesthetic and even an artistic side. Imagine a way to restore facial tissues lost due to injury or disease, in fact, the construction of a new patient's face. No one can deny that this work, firstly, is the handicraft production (performed in a single copy and by hand), and secondly, the art and design solution determines its appearance. What happens if for every picture of his 'art object' the surgeon wants to receive royalties or at least permission to reproduce?

At the moment, these weird questions do not arise because implantable devices are technical objects to which the patient's body has no relation. These objects do not change over time and with the condition of the patient's body, as well as do not grow along with it. At any time, you can pinpoint their presence and localisation; at any time, it is technically possible to remove them (albeit with trauma for the patient) and replace them with a more advanced model. Despite the fact that they are located inside the body, they are foreign bodies. The situation will be changed dramatically after a way will be discovered to place an artificial tissues complex inside the patient's body combined with techno-biological objects, which will be adopted by the body, modified by the patient's body, becoming what they were not at the time of the operation, i.e. grow with the patient in response to the state of patient's health or his nervous system. To a large extent or even fully, they will become an integral part of the patient's body. Nobody can make an unambiguous statement what was, namely, placed in the patient's body, because the results of such a prosthetics after a while would be impossible to distinguish from the natural state. Such prosthesis generally cannot be removed; moreover, it's impossible to clearly delineate its boundaries in the tissues. Thus, the object of patent protection (invention, utility model, or industrial design) will disappear after some time after implementation, but instead the medical outcomes appear that cannot be clearly predicted and depends on a set of random events. But the factors of patentability cannot simply disappear into space. Is the body of the patient the object of patent protection? For a lawyer, the question is not idle.

Such 'a mass' manipulation of the bodies of patients will yield the appropriate results: Gradually, there is a situation where a part of humanity in the developed world will constantly pay for the right to live, after a certain age, or after undergoing certain medical procedures. Such payments to owners of patents can be a constant expense for an ever-growing part of humanity. The problem is that the payment for the very right to life comes into sharp conflict with the laws of the most developed countries, which state that the right to life does not depend on the level of income. Ways out of this situation are only two: either to create a government's financial structure, which would carry out all the payments on behalf of the citizens with prosthesis, or to limit the right patent, completely eliminating from it all biological objects. Both solutions have advantages and disadvantages.

4. C. Analysers Inside the Human Body.
Who Reads the Values?

Contemporary medicine is known to be based on facts. These facts are more and more numbers describing the state of the patient. Even in cases where a patient's condition cannot be measured on any scale, in evidence is a picture of the object of the disease, i.e. again the digital information. Modern medicine is committed to ensuring that any medical diagnostic solution shall be made only on the basis of objective information, which can be written in the form of the measurement of parameters of the human body. The effectiveness of the doctor's work, again, was evaluated by how the changed body parameter came to the border of normal ranges. Two hundred years ago when a doctor told a colleague, 'Look at my patient X and give your opinions', he was referring to an external examination, direct and instrumental. Today, we hear a phrase in clinics: 'Look at the test results of my patient X and tell your views'. The results of the external examination of the patient are no longer a basis for treatment decisions; they are too subjective, unreliable, and shaky as a basis for conclusions. Even the symptoms of the disease, which are visible externally, are put on some objective scale and then measured, i.e. converted to the numbers, by the modern medicine.

Thus, diagnostic activity becomes a monitoring of the parameters of the patient's body. As yet the initiator, the start of the measurement of these parameters is done by the patient himself; that is, for example, nobody can measure the blood pressure or the patient's body temperature without his permission so that he does not even know about it. Currently, the border between the ordinary citizen and the patient is crossed only at the request of the individual. However, in the near future, the state of all its citizens will be considered as patients by definition, as described in the previous chapters. In such circumstances, the state no longer needs the formal permission for starting the diagnostic activity. This transition is the most important change in the paradigm of the medical activity, from the earliest times. Now, as in ancient times, only the patient initiates the treatment, when he decides it's time to go to the doctor because the disease can no longer be tolerated. And usually, this decision is made too late. Dreams of preventive medicine, until recently, were limited to dreams of mass checkups at which the early stages of diseases would be discovered. These dreams remind us of naive pictures of medieval visionaries, depicting the possible construction of aircraft on muscular thrust and submarines with pedals, i.e. dreams ahead of the available technology and, moreover, that which offers the obviously impracticable technical solutions. *Dreams of preventive medicine are basically impossible to actualise on the technological stage of subjective visual and instrumental medical examinations.*

Technological stage of development of medicine in which the permission for the diagnosis of the patient is required is rapidly coming to an end in front of our eyes. At the spur of the moment, a person is alienated from the right to the decision on the diagnostic measurements of his body; he has rights only to the decision to start proper medical actions. Thousands of people in the world already are living under the continuous monitoring of some parameters of their bodies, and for this monitoring, they pay money. Moreover, they do the work of reading the values with a special device and send it to the authorised physician for data analysis. Telemedical monitoring of patients becomes a routine in developed countries. But the first steps of this technology are already showing the degree of its immaturity:

- The effectiveness of this technology often depends on the discipline of the patient who must periodically read parameters with a wearable device.
- Every act of reading options takes time and requires some skill on the part of the patient; the accuracy of the result depends on many random factors.

- Wearable devices require a power supply and periodic calibration, is often quite cumbersome, prone to breakage, and requires an external channel for data transmission.
- Data transfer channels are the ordinary telephone lines, which are fraught with overloading due this technology being widespread and with a sharp increase in the number of passed parameters.
- If you increase the number of people submitting data and frequency of measurement, a man is knowingly not able to produce even the evaluative analysis of the incoming data stream. It's inevitable when the function of the primary data analysis will be trusted to computers.
- There is a significant percentage of patients who cannot make measurements of parameters, even with special reminders. This, in particular, includes children, persons with established psychiatric diagnoses, and very old people (centenarians). Also, the patient is not available for measurements during sleep, which is about a third of life, and after injury, which would lead to the loss of consciousness.

The next logical step in the development of this technology will be a complete rejection of patient participation in the act of measuring the parameters of his body. For a more objective measurement and to avoid physiological reactions to the very fact of measuring the diagnostician will tend towards the situation when the patient will not even know about the specific moments and frequency of measurements. That is, the transition will be to the hidden measurements and for some easily measurable parameters—to their continuous registration (monitoring). Rather, such a transition will begin with a certain age (children) and professional groups (pilots, vehicle drivers, military personnel), simply because the benefits of using medical monitoring of these groups are much more obvious, and it is much more easier to get funding for such the tasks.

Specific details of this technology are difficult to predict; we can only speak of individual principles and approaches. First of all, in the early stages they will create a closed habitat, which for a long time have to live the object of observation. It can include pre-schools, schools, recreation centres, children's hospitals, orphanages. In such institutions, they can create a specific environment, saturated with hidden sensors for remote or contact monitoring of an ever-expanding range of parameters of the human body. It is possible that the measurements will be performed as well and at night when it is technically convenient to measure some of the parameters, using the fact that the child is asleep at immobility and his brain does not react to the fact of the measurement itself. The next place to monitor the health of patients may be a military object, the staff of which is isolated for a long time; in particular, such patients can become the operators of weapons systems that are on constant alert, crews of submarines, surface ships, aircrafts, and command posts. It is known that the crews of space ships and space stations since the beginning of manned space flights were objects of remote medical monitoring.

As the technologies of hidden measurements of the human body will become simpler and cheaper, they will spread to all humanity. At first, the 'tracking' will be at job places, then the places of commercial leisure (resorts, hotels, clubs), and then residences (apartments, houses). The presence of environment that monitors the patients will be the most important safety factor in this particular environment, and the mankind is never spared any expense on safety. You can anticipate the evolving of the laws when obliging owners equip the living space with such systems; just as they now have to install security and fire systems, the emergency rooms in public places should be maintained. There will be a gradual transition to the creation of a universal, friendly living environment, which keeps track of all beings in it, members of the species Homo sapiens. This habitat is a *completely new tool for collecting data on the human population* as a whole, namely, the following:

- First and most obvious is that such an environment knows the number of observed objects and at any given time up to one person. Moreover, the system knows the surnames' list of objects of observation. Population census has become an amusing anachronism. Absolutely accurate knowledge of the structure of the population in the given time will immediately affect the quality of planning of the production of goods and services, in particular, social and medical.
- This environment will be able to detect the mass diseases (epidemics) at a very early stage of development, simply by grouping similar symptoms in a number of patients registered in a particular area for a short period of time. Most importantly, all the objective data will be known to the system even before the mass conversion of patients to the doctor. Such assistance will raise the anti-epidemic services to a whole new level; in particular, the system can 'seek out' the patients with specific symptoms or a combination of them in the huge mass of people and do it constantly.
- The system can monitor a particular patient, his relatives, or any group (statistical sampling) of the patients that are of interest to social and medical research. Thus, studies that are now produced with the participation of volunteers and paid for in money in the future often will be carried out very quickly and cheaply, without distracting patients from their usual life and, in certain circumstances, even without their knowledge. The humanity will obtain a powerful tool for a completely new type of scientific researches of himself, to automatically receive the social and medical

data on the population with almost no human labour costs and time.

- Such a system will optionally record the variations in the health status of certain groups in certain situations, such as during and after the using of certain transport, visiting certain places, living in certain environments, and feeding on certain foods. The information may be a key in assessing the benefits and harms caused by certain circumstances of life, followed by recommendations for change in the place and lifestyle. It is particularly important that such information will be extracted automatically and very cheaply and be statistically significant based on the huge amount of data (can being used to assess 100% of the target audience and not to use the statistical sampling).

- Demography as a science goes to a whole new level. Now one can assess changes in the structure of society as a whole and in individual arbitrarily narrow groups in real time and up to one person. So, it can predict the structure of the population in the future with a very high accuracy.

- Emergency care systems will receive a reliable automatic assistant that will advise them on critical medical situations at the moment of occurrence, even if the victim is alone and unconscious. This warning system will radically reduce the mortality due to emergency and mass trauma, especially when you consider that health workers that go on a call will know in advance the number and age of the victims, as well as the nature and severity of the injury.

- Such a system some time after the start of the operation becomes a kind of 'time machine'; that is, at any time the historical data may be requested. For example, the system will definitely answer the question: 'What were the numbers of average arterial blood pressure in females over 55 years old, living permanently in the given area three years ago in the period from September to December?'. Today even asking such a question does not make sense.

- The system can monitor the effectiveness of the operation of new artificial organs and bioimplants were described in the previous chapter. At some stage, the bionic implant (prosthesis) itself can be a reprogrammable universal organ of the body to allow the organism to communicate with their environment; that is, technology of bionic prosthetics and intracorporeal tracking the status of the body will merge into one.

With the development of the technology of miniaturisation will become clear that it's the technologically beneficial for measuring the device and the sensor (a) inside the patient's body and (b) which is available for the prophylaxis or replacement. That is, there will be transition to the intracorporeal analysers, i.e. those that are inside the body.

The chain of data transmission can be arranged based on the client-server technology and as the server will serve namely the intracorporeal device that responds to requests from the environment in the standard way: by passing its individual ID and number characterising the measured value, but the clients are the wireless sensors, scattered in the environment and associated with database. After receiving the patient data, they are supplemented by the exact date and time of receipt and sent to the centre for primary analysis. Convenience will be primarily in the fact that intracorporeal microsensors will not require power, as it will be powered by the energy of the body in one form or another. It will be of great convenience that the patient may not lose his sensor, spoil it, mix up it with someone else's sensor; in addition, the patient can maintain his usual way of life by swimming, playing water sports, or working in a chemically aggressive environment. The expansion of support of such technology can be simply by placing an increasing number of devices-clients for all the new territories and habitats and increasing their action radius; the intracorporeal devices themselves will not require intervention except when they will be replaced by the more advanced device, which measures more parameters with greater accuracy.

The advantages of a living habitat, organised this way, we can list in a long time, but the medic-technologist would be primarily interested in the question and what will be its dangers and disadvantages. The first and main danger I see is much more access to the personal data of patients-citizens and also to the very intimate data about their health. Also, there is the danger of using the system to spy on its citizens by state. It is time now to try to answer the question posed in the title of the chapter: 'Who takes the information?'

That the information is automatically collected should not deceive us. First, the sensor-server while responding to client requests cannot know whether the device is authorised by the client to ask him. Second, the data will inevitably pass through the nodes of the network that in principle are available for hacking. And third, the central database itself with backups is a small titbit to crack. That is, they have to solve some intricate problems to protect the data of patients. Here we must say a few things:

- Humanity changes its attitudes to security, especially as to which information is secret and which is not. Only a few hundred years ago, the most important state secrets were the number of troops and weapons, horses and fighting ships, waterways and coastlines, castle plans and time passwords. Today, no one cares for this, and what is the meaning to hide what is visible to anyone who has access to the orbiting satellites? From today's perspective, the most important state secrets are an effective weapon technology and technology (access) of its management. From the perspective of future, the health issues of a particular patient may completely cease to be interesting to anyone other than himself, his doctor, and family members.

- Fully able to make that the process of abduction (reading), the data of patients by unauthorised users become very time-consuming and useless from the point of view of mass accumulation of data, for example, to provide the individual data encryption. That is, each sensor transmits its data using his own code, then the data is transmitted in the undeciphered form and in the same form will be placed in a central database. Only authorised users with access to a central database can see the decrypted data. Protection of encryption keys on this level is a much more easy thing. In this approach, the mass abduction of user data will be incredibly time-consuming (and therefore economically unfavourable) process; in addition, the stolen data will reflect only the current time, which drastically reduces their value.

- Organisation with access to the decrypted patient database cannot be a business; it is a matter of national security. The fact is that even depersonalised data on all patients in the country are huge, a key value for the players in the market. Such information could be very valuable for investigations of hostile states. Information about the growth or, conversely, the reduction in the number of people suffering from certain medical conditions or who are the carriers of certain medical problems (even if they do not know about it) is the input for the far-reaching marketing moves in multiple markets.

Such a summary of the information of public health should belong to a society as a whole, i.e. a public organisation with several degrees of social control, which could give it in doses only to people who prove the need for it, for example, scientists engaged in research in the field of public health, sanitation, epidemiology, demography, etc. At the same time, information about a specific patient and his relatives is the subject of the working interest of a particular doctor, who should have access to it while performing official duties. But the fact is that even a non-poor public organisation cannot create and maintain the extensive and very expensive resource base for the operation of such a living environment; this can be done only by the state. Thus, we are speaking about the organisation with a fairly specific status: resource base created and maintained by the authority of the state on the tax money, but the owner and manager of the data in such a system is a public organisation.

4. D. Individual Medications and Modulators. Who Is Responsible for the Outcome of Treatment?

It is known that the pharmacology as the science about interaction of substances with living organisms was born in the Middle Ages and that its founders were not doctors but alchemists that continuously operated with retorts and the very strange substances from which they were trying to retrieve the Philosopher's Stone. Namely, the alchemists were first exposed to substances that were produced in their retorts; sometimes it cost health and life. Even then, it was observed that the chemicals had different effects on different people. In particular, it was clearly manifested in attempts of preparation and application of various poisons, which involved a good deal of practical skills of any alchemist and later pharmacists, who gradually shifted from the use of herbs to the use of chemistry. To standardise the methods of preparing, names of medicines have been issued in special documents, later called pharmacopoeias. The first such document appeared in the ninth century in Arab countries; much later, such documents appeared in Europe (fifteenth to seventeenth centuries).

Pharmacopeia had established the national standards of medications, which greatly simplified their manufacture and use. Also, the training of future doctors and pharmacists was simplified. But after the standardisation of medications used, issues that were previously masked by the disorder in the apothecary techniques came to the fore: *one and the same medication at the same dose acted in different degrees for different people.* Moreover, sometimes there were people in whom some medications (including the poisons) did not have an effect at all or they were affected but not like the others.

They began experimenting with the dosage of the medications, and interesting things came to light: It seemed that it was *impossible to predict unequivocally the effect of the medication at a given dose for a given individual*; we can only talk about the probability of a typical reaction to this medication. Generally, the word 'probability' is too frequently used in this book, is it not? Based on the severity of the reaction of the organism to the amount of active substance, the modern pharmacology distinguishes between the following:

- *The threshold or minimum effective dose*—amount of substance on the introduction of which the majority of patients show a basic biological effect.
- *The median therapeutic dose*—the amount of substance on the introduction of which the majority of patients show the expected pharmacotherapeutic effect.
- *The maximum therapeutic dose*—the amount of substance the introduction of which is safe for most of patients.
- *Toxic dose*—amount of substance that causes the majority of patients to have toxic effects.
- *Lethal dose*—the amount of matter the introduction of which causes death of the majority of patients.

Thus, it turned out that all of the above doses for different people are different. With the current accuracy, it is quite difficult to find two people who would react exactly the same to the same dose of the same factory lot of medication. It was found that some drugs due to its mechanism of action cannot simply be given a dose in grams, like the others, it is necessary to dose them per unit of body weight and some even by body surface area (i.e. m^2). There are even drugs that are dosed in pharmacological international units (IU), i.e. their activity is determined by experiments on biological objects. This biological standardisation is used for medications, for which the exact structure of the active substance is unknown or chemical methods are insufficient for standardisation.

In addition to the clear differences in the doses to people of all age groups, it became clear that there are also the gender and even the racial differences in reactions to pharmaceuticals. The reason for these differences is often hidden in the structure of a single gene. By the way, this proves once again that even minor genetic changes can lead to serious consequences in the body's response to drugs. Doctors now think about the fact that before using the 'serious' medications the genetic testing of patients should be carried out. This selection will identify those most sensitive to the medication, and, of course, those for whom the application of the drug can be dangerous.

We cannot make our bodies identical by definition; these differences allow us to be individuals, or rather, our unique identity is a consequence of the fact that our bodies are different. Thus, the pursuit of efficiency of pharmaceutical remedies will lead to the fact that in the near future we can expect not only a process of individualisation of drug dosage and mode of its administration but also their exact composition and even the design of the dosage form. In particular, differentiation may be subject to the following:

- The proportions of the active ingredients in the dosage form, if more than one.
- Introduction of the unusual active substances to the dosage form to which the patient has an individual sensitivity.
- Introduction or removal of the ballast from the dosage form or forming substances to which the patient has an individual sensitivity.
- Significant changes in the configuration of the molecules of the active substance or the inclusion of the substances-transporters so they will be better able to penetrate biological barriers of the body of the given patient.
- Changes in the active substance's molecules for intentionally creating a depot in certain tissues and organs in the elimination pathways of the medications.

- Changes in the active substance's molecules for subsequent detection of their accumulation in the tissues by modern imaging techniques, which can be a valuable diagnostic information.

Thus, a gradual *abandonment of the concept of mass production of finished products 'for all' in favour of the concept of the production of personalised medicines* for narrow target groups of patients, as well as the production of 'pharmaceutical half-stuff,' designed to reworking in specialised pharmacies, may happen in the pharmaceutical industry. The scheme of relations between the physician and the pharmacist can get back to a medieval version, when a doctor writes a prescription for the pharmacist who prepares the individual medication for the individual patient. But at a given stage of pharmtechnology, the recipe can consist not of a mixture of the active ingredients in given proportions but in the changing of the structure (modifications) of the active substance's molecules for the individual treatment of the medical conditions in this patient. The effectiveness of this approach to medicamentous therapy may be significantly higher than the current one.

It is possible to predict the beginning of the massive use of substances-modulators which have no direct therapeutic action, but change the properties of certain tissues, membranes, organelles, or individual cells so that they acquire new properties, both in terms of resistance to damaging factors and in terms of specific individual benefits for the patient. In particular, such modulators will be popular after the implementation of technologies of bionic prosthetic organs, when there is a need to quickly switch on and off its individual modules or put them into specific mode of operation.

Even today, effective pharmacotherapy is an intricate task for the physician. When selecting the type of the active substance, its dosage, and dose frequency, the future doctor will have to consider a lot of countervailing factors affecting the outcome of treatment:

- Gender and race of patient;
- Other medications and modulators of conditions are taken constantly;
- Substances that fall into the patient through the skin with cosmetics and detergents;
- Substances that enter the body with food and drink (especially food additives, dyes, tonics);
- Features of the physical activity and drinking regimen of the patient, which may affect the rate of excretion of the active substance from the body;
- The history of using pharmacological substances with a similar chemical structure for the given patient;
- Features the immune system of the patient, individual sensitivity to substances defined by class, the history of vaccination.

Accounting for such a huge number of factors without the use of computer technology is problematic even today. The whole question is not how to take them into account, but how to collect them. Modern human often has no idea what namely enters into his body through food, beverages, and cosmetics and thoughtlessly takes vitamin preparations. It's useless asking the patient about this; it's much more effective to take the analysis of relevant biological fluids of his body. Of course, for such an analysis, it requires a very special type of equipment that can detect the presence of a vast range of chemical species (and their decay products) in trace amounts. In fact, we are talking about an intellectual automated chemical laboratory, capable of taking a small sample of blood or tissue to determine the full set of foreign chemicals that enter the body in recent times. Such a device is the dream of a modern doctor and, in particular, the medical examiner. If there is any such evidence, the doctor of the future will be able to accurately correct the individual dose of medication, dosage form, individual dose frequency, and even the exact configuration of molecules of a substance capable of getting to the target organ of the patient. If necessary, the substance-transporter can be injected in the composition of the medication to facilitate the penetration of medication through biological membranes of the given patient.

The schedule for implementation of these technologies will depend heavily on technology of implementation in the intellectual's living environment, as described in the previous chapter. With permanent residence in the environment in which there is no chance to develop any of the disease to such an extent that requires serious pharmacotherapy; the above described high-tech ways of drugs' customisation may be too expensive to implement. There is a question of comparative costs of these two technologies in the society. A technology that will be implemented first will suppress the appearance of the another. Watching the current rate of development of microelectronics and computer networks, it seems to me that the creation of an intellectual living environment will overtake the development of customised medications. But in case of a sudden breakthrough in nanotechnology, all could change.

In the case of the scenario of customised pharmacotherapy in all growth, the legal issue of the division of responsibility for the outcome of treatment will rise. As involvement in the treatment process of a growing number of medical experts, the process of division of responsibility for the overall outcome is becoming more and more unfair. If you recall the situation of a century ago, the doctor then was indeed solely responsible for the outcome. The doctor did himself all analyses of his patient; he counted the blood cells in a smear. (Do you remember the required microscope on the physician's desktop in the photographs of the early twentieth century?) He himself would look for infectious agents in smears of patient's biological fluids; he himself did the urine tests for sugar and much more. The doctor himself did all more or less complex manipulations at the bedside of the patient, including injections and dressing; a nurse at the time was more like an attendant. In those days, if the patient told that he was treated by a doctor X, it was so. Now if a patient says that he is treated in hospital X, he's right. The responsibility of one doctor for the overall outcome becomes a legal formality; it's just easier for the justice system.

In fact, the physician can no longer be solely responsible for the overall result, as most of the treatment decisions he takes on the basis of alien information obtained by other health professionals: specialty-related doctors, laboratory technicians, radiologists, nurses, technicians for maintenance of diagnostic equipment, social workers, and even the police. The modern physician is also highly dependent on the quality of the pharmaceuticals. In the evolution of technology of customised pharmaceutical production, further dissipation of responsibility will happen for the final medical outcome between the manufacturers of pharmaceutical semi-automated diagnosing biochemical laboratories, specialists in calibration and maintenance of the equipment, apparatus for drugs' customisation, doctors which prescribed the medication, and the patients who were forced to take a customised medication by a certain and rather rigid scheme.

Questions of legal responsibility for treatment failure will be very inconvenient for practical use; they will be forced to subpoena a few dozen experts immediately. It will be easier to break the whole process of treatment into individual fragments that are available for reliable quality control and assign the responsible professionals for each stage. In such circumstances, for the patient's lawsuit they will have to address not a doctor or even a clinic in general but the particular specialist that is responsible for the outcome of a particular link in the technological chain. In the medical law, there will be a new specialisation: advising on the proper filing of claims for treatment failure associated with the identification of the part of the technological chain in which the failure occurred, and not the fact that this part will be located in the hospital. That is, identification of the failed link will be taken outside of the trial and will be up to the court. This is a very difficult task for now, and the situation will only become more complex.

If we consider pharmacotherapy as repair of the human body that in many ways still is a 'black box' for us, because we often still do not fully understand what exactly caused this or that pharmacological effect, there will be a more progressive concept of refusal of repair of tissues body in favour of a replacement of defective individual tissues and whole organs of the body. In fact, if you look at how humanity repairs less and less things around and replaces more and more the defective items with new ones which are more progressive and useful, would not it be more logical to replace the tissues? Recently, progress has accelerated so much that things, clothes, shoes, appliances are being replaced with new ones, even if the old can still work; that is, *timing of introduction of new technologies become shorter than the service life of products made on old technology*. Nothing prevents from the same process beginning in medicine. In the next chapter, we will talk about the consequences that may result in the introduction of controlled regeneration of human tissues.

4. E. Driven Tissue Regeneration. No More Disability?

The fact that the lesions heal was known even to the cave-dwellers. They were also aware that the lost segments of the limbs and organs of a person could not be restored, as opposed to, say, newts and lizards. Loss of one limb in prehistoric and ancient times was a huge loss, and if the man did not belong to the elite class, it meant that he could not fully work and hunt, and in many cases it was death by starvation. Persons who had lost two limbs at once were a great rarity in the age of lack of mechanical transportation and machinery and rarely survived due to the severity of such an injury. The number of amputees increased dramatically just in the beginning of the era of mass application of firearms (injured with cannonball, shrapnel, the mine blast injuries), mechanical transport and machines, as well as owing to advances in surgical technique of amputation. Namely, a huge number of amputees after every major war has led many developed countries to the idea of a system of universal pensions. The word 'pensioner' originally meant a former soldier who was unable to work because of the wounds of war and got the content out of the treasury. Military pensioners first appeared in ancient Rome under Julius Caesar; civil pensioners appeared much later. Pension systems that cover the entire population of the country had appeared only by the early twentieth century; the pioneers in this field were Germany (1889), Denmark (1891), and New Zealand (1898).

The modern tendency to preserve the patient's limb at every small opportunity and fight for every inch of stump for better prosthetics afterwards was not just an illustration of the increased capabilities of surgeons and a common desire for humanity. The current pension system of developed states is the motor development of these technologies and the conductor of the new social maxim: *the health care system should not produce new disabilities.* Pension funds of states that crack under the pressure of new pensioners, generations of which are far more numerous than they were fifty years ago, stimulate the health care of their countries for the immediate implementation of technologies for preservation workability, even if limited or even formal.

Under conditions of threat of the collapse of the pension systems in the developed countries, there are not too many options for survival in the social protection systems:

1. The easiest way to solve a problem is administrative: Just push ahead the retirement age, at least for the most numerous categories of new retirees. In developed countries with a high life expectancy, this method does not actually cure the problem, but pushes it ahead, giving the social security system a few years of respite per basic change in production technologies with improved productivity, which also based on the sharp progress in treatment of elderly and disabled people and their socialisation. In underdeveloped countries with a low life expectancy, this solution really cures the problem due to the fact that most old people simply do not live up to the new retirement age. But to the extent that a country develops and life expectancy grows, the problem will come back at any age of retirement. Thus, the simplest ways to solve in this case do not work.

2. The development of labour markets, specially adapted for specific categories of pensioners and people with disabilities, along with appearance of new jobs and professions, adapted to the needs and opportunities of citizens with disabilities. The idea is not new and is already being implemented in many developed countries.

3. Breakthrough in the treatment of injuries and diseases that cause disability, controlled regeneration of human tissues, developing new ways of socialising peoples with

disabilities, advanced prosthetics of lost organs and its individual functions.

4. Comprehensive development of private pension systems and corporate social protection systems that remove the part of the load from the state.

We are interested primarily in the third point, namely, *medical methods* of preventing the onset of disability. This refers to the most common causes of disability: loss of limbs, injuries, and diseases of the internal organs (especially the heart and large vessels) and injuries and diseases of the senses (sight and hearing). Investment in research to develop a controlled regeneration of certain types of tissues and then whole bodies seem to me the most effective way to remove most of the load in the future social protection systems. Nobody can foresee in which particular area the first scientific breakthrough will happen, but governments, corporations, and civil society organisations are logically investing in those areas that can provide the most economic benefits.

The discovery of a way to control the regeneration of certain tissues may lead to effects that the developers and investors are not counted upon, for example, increasing the degree of social injustice in the determination of the applicability of such medical technologies. Imagine that the technology of 'growing' a new limb directly on the stump of the patient will be reliably implemented only for younger age cohorts of patients. The state will eventually have to draw somewhere the age limit of applicability of this technology, as well as the insurance companies will need to respond to tough questions of patients and relatives why state pays for such treatment of a person, say, five years old, and does not pay for the same treatment at the age of six years. Social tension between generations, which exists now, may further increase. Even more uncomfortable questions may arise, if it turns out that the application of these technologies is associated with the patient's gender, that is, available to one gender and completely inaccessible to another. Generally speaking, to the extent that as medical technologies will become 'thinner' and work on the level of cellular molecular mechanisms, the likelihood that some vital technology will not be available for a portion of the human population due to minor differences in the genotype will increase.

Another aspect of injustice associated with the introduction of such a technology is related to its cost. At a very high initial cost, as is usually the case with new technology, it will benefit individual disabled people with very high income or people in the very rich countries, which governments can invest heavily in its population. Such persons with disabilities are present only in developed countries with a high per capita income. Thus, the countries will immediately be divided into those where the technology is applied and those where it is not at all, as there are no paying customers. This situation will give more economic opportunities to developed countries and further strengthen the lag of developing countries.

Social and health consequences of the introduction of controlled tissue regeneration are rather hard to imagine. Many medical professions will change dramatically so that the doctors will have to completely retrain because the very paradigm of the doctor's actions will change. In fact, why spend the time, efforts, and money on expensive hospital treatment of severe fractures or bone tumour, if you can immediately perform minimal amputation after it to grow a new limb for the patient? The same goes for orthopaedic pathology, vascular diseases of extremities, and effects of trauma and burns. The whole question is the comparative cost of such a hypothetical technology as against conventional treatment. As the cost of this technology becomes lower, most of modern traumatology and orthopaedics and partially the vascular surgery will be permanently abandoned. Also the combustiology will be completely changed, while the opportunities to grow up the skin flap of any form and area for the patient with burns will arise. Also, plastic surgery will be completely different. This technology will change the consciousness of the doctor so much that most will not be able to retrain until the end of their life. The situation will resemble the appearance of antibiotics; many doctors will not change his mind, i.e. formally recognising the benefit of antibiotics, but themselves will work the old way, without them. And only the new generation of doctors will be able to fully use them. It is easy to predict also some abuse of new technologies in the initial period, using them without indications in the same way as it was the case when revolutionary antibiotics appeared in the 1950s of the last century, and the young doctors prescribe them even in cases where their use can be easily avoided.

The next logical step of this technology will be growing up the entire organs for patients; this can be done beforehand, and the question is the cost of cultivation and storage of such products. Nothing prevents the heart from growing up in advance (liver, kidney, pancreas) for the patient and to keep it up to a certain age. Cardiology and nephrology under such conditions have completely changed and in fact will be the technologies of tracking the time when the heart or kidney can be transplanted in the patient (i.e. economically rational). If this technology is implemented, then at some point it may be worth less than the traditional treatment of the patient's organ. In this case, the treatment technologies could be very quickly (within a generation of doctors) discarded as being economically inefficient and will be replaced by technology of the driven regeneration of organs. Many medical specialties, sadly, will disappear quite as almost the repair experts of clothes and shoes have disappeared: People just prefer to buy new goods, because they are much better (and sometimes even cheaper) than older ones.

However, the problem already described in the previous chapters appears: the question of the ownership of such grown (cloned) organs. Given that it is grown from the patient's own tissues, it is necessary to decide a legal question. What does the involved company do: the fabrication of the bio-product to sell or servicing the patient, consisting of the fact that they allow the patient's cells to grow and multiply in a supportive environment for them? In any case, private banks of organs will be a very profitable and popular business, as a rare patient does not want to have their spare organs in case of injury or illness. Donation of organs and tissues, as we know it today, will disappear quickly as economically ruinous, because alien organs will require preliminary and very expensive procedures of tissue typing. But the transplantation surgery will be one of the most popular medical specialties in the future.

These will not be without legal consequences. In particular, it could change the legal definition of the terms 'bodily injury' and 'damage to health'. In the future, the loss of the upper extremity as a result of damage in developed countries will be described by the words 'injury, which led to temporary disability,' and loss of an eye will be qualified as 'minor injuries, accompanied by moral suffering'. In medicine, a strange mass diagnosis such as 're-cirrhosis' or 're-glomerulonephritis' will appear—the disease of the transplanted liver or kidney. The next chapter will address the question of whether it is possible to variegate artificially the human population at the early stage of embryo development and whether mankind wants to be diverse.

4. F. In Vitro Fertilisation with Genetic Control. The Artificial Variety of Populations?

If an early medieval man would now walk the streets of any European capital city, he will be impressed by not just the height of buildings, advertising, cleanliness of streets, and street traffic. No less, he will be struck by a variety of individuals, height growth, shades of skin colours, and diversity of clothes and hairstyles of our contemporaries. Mankind has become much more diverse in every single point of residence, even in comparison with the situation of a century ago, and it's not just a matter of clothes. Our contemporaries are paying money to make a tattoo in a visible place, pierce themselves with something to put jewellery there, or make an incredible hairstyle. Cosmetics of residents of developed countries often resembles the war paint of African tribes. There are already even more advanced people, which have implanted the electronic chips under their skin for various purposes. Question is whether it is just fashion for embellishment, which will soon pass, or an internal human need for individual variation of the body, on the realisation of resources and capabilities which previously were not available.

It depends on the correct answer to this question, I think. Before our eyes, there is a huge new market and its size is comparable to the modern fashion industry and cosmetics. For now it is at the children's stage of body piercing and tattoo studios, but as they will mature, they will be interested in serious market players and serious investors. First of all, we should understand the extent to which mankind would like to be diverse. Does this needs changing over time?

It seems to me that this question falls in the set of problems. Man wants to be beautiful not only in his own eyes but also, above all, in the eyes of others. If in the community there's a long-term tendency to call 'beautiful' (and therefore 'functional') this or that the external quality of man, the majority of people in the population will try to fit in this concept. When we change the concept of beautiful in this society, the fashion on appearance changes as well. The whole question is *at what velocity*. If the concept of beautiful changes rapidly, man could be limited by a change of clothes, shoes, and hairstyles. With a slower change in fashion, that is comparable to the time of life for generations—changes begin to relate also to the human body. If we recall how the European women looked in the times of Rubens (only 400 years ago), today we would consider all of them as obese, but they considered themselves beautiful. And vice versa, today's mannequins would consider the times of Rubens as one step away from starvation. The reason for these changes is long-term (more than a hundred years) women's fashion for the thin waist. The last several generations of women were 'on a diet'. People were willing to put up with any inconvenience and even endure physical pain (women's and men's corsets) just to meet the fashion on appearance. It is now difficult to know where this fashion started, but it is clearly supported by explicit efforts of leading players in the world of fashion, and they can be understood: For the standard figure it is easier to sew. So the first problem is the *velocity of changes in the appearance*, namely, the longer the presence of any fashion, the deeper the people allow to change their appearance, gradually getting used to it. At some stage, it inevitably begins to change the human body itself.

The second problem is the *changing of the concept of 'healthy person' and, in particular, the concept of 'healthy baby'.* If 300 years ago, they asked the average mother about the child she wanted, most of all, she would answer simply and briefly: 'healthy'. The notion of a 'healthy child' then meant 'like everybody and who survives'. Today the requirements of the mother are much more complex: She not only wants a surviving child but also that she (he) has the appearance of a movie star, not below average intelligence, is an athlete, can swim, dance, know foreign languages, plays music, and has an artistic taste . . . no sickness (even childhood infections), no hereditary diseases that he would give to his grandchildren; the growth should be above average, have a good eyesight and hearing, even in old age, and she (he) should have a healthy digestion, thus she would not have to limit herself to food and have healthy teeth lifelong, etc., etc. Today the demands of parents for appearance, intelligence, and level of health in their children have become much more varied and more severe than it was recently. Some parents already want to choose the eye and hair colour for their children. And note that many of these requirements are addressed to the doctors, and it is not surprisingly, since the parents get their child from a man in a white coat. The fact that now almost children who are born survive leads to a natural result: Humanity is becoming more diverse in terms of health. Despite the ever-increasing level of expectations of the parents, their children are more divergent in terms of compliance with this health level. Their standard of living (of course, I'm talking about the developed countries with high social standards) is less and less dependent on the health level and physical conditions and more and more on the creativity, workability, and intelligence. Thus, in social consciousness there's a mismatch: There is on the one hand, all the more rigid boundaries of the concept of 'healthy person', arising to the extent that an increasing number of parameters of the human body is made available for the measurement, while on the other hand, even more wider range of medical conditions in the population living in all countries now. It leads to the situation when the percentage of the population that can be officially recognised as healthy all the time is reduced, which creates a clear but false impression of the population that the physicians and the health system as a whole are getting worse and worse to cope with their work.

To get out of this situation, in my opinion, it is possible only in one way: to recognise that the concept of a 'healthy person' currently is strongly narrowed, which, in turn, means that *many of the people we now consider as sick really are healthy, but they're healthy 'differently*, for their life's circumstances, their lifestyles, and for their environment. This is a very significant process from the point of view of the mass consciousness of humanity: On the one hand, it is known that all people are equal in their rights, while on the other hand, the mankind is clearly beginning to be variable in appearance and the parameters of their body. It is very important to humanity that it at once cements that fact in its consciousness and in the law, otherwise the rollback from the policy of equal rights regardless of the structure of the body and their health level may happen.

Realisation of the fact that humanity becomes nonuniform and divided into some subspecies, depending on the structure of the body, the characteristics of metabolism, the milestone modernisations of the body, the degree of longevity, and some parameters of the body, resulting in significant differences in the ability to work and social communication, will cause the long adjustment period, but it will be incomparably shorter than the adaptation of medieval man to the fact that the American Indian, Eskimo, or Australian Aborigine is the same man as he was, but only adapted to different habitats (at that time it took a few centuries). Globalisation will further speed up the process.

Over time, most of the governments will have a simple idea: People do not need to adapt to the environments. It is economically more efficient and more humane to do the opposite: create habitats that are pre-adapted to the needs and characteristics of the body structure of separate subspecies of humanity. As technology of bionic prosthetic of bodies and their individual functions, these two technologies will come together: People will be born pre-adapted under the environments specially designed for them. What are these new living environments we cannot know in advance; it will be solved by the residents themselves: It is possible that at first the difference in air pressure, atmospheric composition, temperature and humidity, the presence of various types of radiation, etc. will be discussed. With the accumulation of differences in the structure of bodies and its physiology, the housing environment with much more significant differences can be designed.

When these specific living environments will be many, and therefore, the differences of people living in them, we will understand the fact that ensuring the conformity of the human organism and its habitat is more convenient and cheaper, namely at a stage of embryonic development. Many embryos at different stages of their development and with the consent of their biological parents will undergo a chain of meaningful manipulations, leading to their adaptation to the specific living environment. Of course, not all parents will agree with this practice; we can predict the emergence of social and religious movements that oppose any interference in the human body. In any case, humanity will be gradually divided into two subspecies: 'adapted' and 'universal', i.e. natural. And that those and others will have their advantages and limitations. 'Natural' people can be proud of its versatility and ability to live in a natural environment, being exposed to the harmful effects of man-made emissions and pollutions. When visiting the artificial environments they will use certain safety equipment. In contrast, the 'adapted' people can comfortably and for a long time live and work in their artificial habitat, but when visiting the other artificial environments, as well as the natural living environment, they will be forced to use special means of protection. In general, *some part of mankind can exchange the freedom of living in any of the natural environment of the planet with the quality and duration of life in an artificial environment.*

Thus, mankind will proceed to the artificial diversity of the human population, which will mark a new stage in its evolutionary development. Unlike earlier, this stage will be completely man-made. At some stage, there will appear as different types of human organisms. In a famous novel *'The Time Machine'*, written in the eve of the twentieth century, in 1895, H.G. Wells described a division of humanity in the very distant future (he pointed to the year 802,701) into two branches as a result of natural evolutionary processes. I think that the division of mankind into many subspecies can occur much faster (by the standards of evolution—tomorrow) and in an artificial way, from considerations of the benefits of adaptation to the environments. Such an extension of the concept of 'man' cannot occur without changes in the law. As we remember, at some point, the developed countries were forced to write in the Constitution that the rights of people does not depend on race and gender. What will be written in the future law in the determining of the human being? We'll discuss this in the next chapter.

4. G. Legal Implications: Fragmentation of Health Law Field for People of Different Types?

Rudiments of health law can be found in the earliest written laws of mankind. People from ancient times tried to set the rules that had to do with one who treats and the one who was treated. These regulations were like the cast of morality at those times. As soon as the morals of society started changing, the rules of behaviour of physicians and patients started to immediately change as well. What's interesting is the causes of the need to regulate the behaviour of the subjects of the medical activities of people are gradually changing over time:

- Initially, the cause of the rules of conduct of doctors were huge losses because of charlatans' activity, which the patients in those days could not distinguish from the doctors, because then there were no diploma. Complaints usually were sent to the highest level of government, which tried to solve the problems in its characteristic way. Primarily, they were interested in the opportunity to take revenge for the failure of medical treatment or even the death of a relative, as well as to curb the doctors' attempts to artificially inflate the prices of their services. The Code of the Babylonian king *Hammurabi* in 1780 BC even called for the specific amounts of fines that must be paid by the doctor for unsuccessful treatment, as well as the amount of payment for certain medical manipulations; in particular, Section 218 of the Code of *Hammurabi* says: 'If a physician make a large incision with the operating knife, and kill him, or open a tumour with the operating knife, and cut out the eye, his hand shall be cut off.' According to Section 221 of the Code of *Hammurabi*, 'If a physician heal the broken bone or diseased soft part of a man, the patient shall pay the physician five shekels in money.' This amount could feed a few people for a whole year. That is, these laws standardised the behaviour of physicians and patients from an economic point of view (the issues of payment services and compensation for the failure and the damage). In those days, medical services were not different from the usual purchase and sale.

- In ancient times, the rules of conduct of doctors also began to regulate the different vows, which brought the graduates of different medical schools-clans. It was a kind of internal corporate code of conduct aimed at closing the medical knowledge of the society, with a list of unlawful methods of healing, allowing to receive compensation without successful treatment, as well as examples of unacceptable behaviour of the doctor in terms of morality of the time. One of these was the famous Oath of *Hippocrates*; thanks to the representatives of Kos school that it was recorded. These vows were more like statutes of secret societies and could not regulate the relations of the quite closed medical community to the outside world. It was a time of free medical merchants who fought for the most revenue in the unregulated market of medical services.

- In the Middle Ages, the code of conduct of European medicals was entirely within the Christian morality; that is, all that was approved by the Church was considered appropriate in the behaviour of the doctor and patient, and on the contrary, all that went beyond Christian morality was suppressed. However, at that time the beginnings of modern medical law in terms of the *admission of physicians in the market* started to appear—the formal medical diplomas came in importance, resembling today's medical license to practice. The doctor-patient relationship is still reminiscent of the transaction of purchase and sale with the formal right to sue for fraud, which may prove to be the doctor and the patient. The intra-corporative laws direct their main efforts to the correct section of the market of considerably grown medical services and to prevent the spreading of medical knowledge into the hands of the uninitiated.

- Medical law in the modern sense of the word appears in the developed countries, only during the formation of early health systems (late nineteenth century) because between the patient and doctor the state appears for the first time with other interests than the interests of the patient and the doctor. Namely, the work of the state to find a balance between all the participants in health and social processes leads to a fundamentally new branch of law, which was not in the classical Roman law, nor in the Civil Code of *Napoleon*. This section describes the *rules by which the given society reached agreement to control its quantity, longevity, and level of health*. The human society in its history has not experienced such needs before.

- In today's world, the medical technology is progressing so rapidly that public opinion does not have time to develop a new attitude for them, which could satisfy the majority of the population and express it in the new legislation. As the result, the unified medical legal space 'breaks'; gaps appear in relation to which the developed countries are waging a fierce controversy. This leads to fundamentally different approaches to certain specific issues of medical law in different countries, which begins to significantly affect the proliferation of new medical technologies as well as the physicians who use them. Medical law in the world is no longer completely homogeneous. This is a very important process, because the *heterogeneous medical legislation will eventually produces the heterogeneity of the population.*

- In the near future, the separation processes of medical law on the enclaves will get further logical development, since there is no indication that the rate of introduction of new medical technologies is diminishing. On the contrary, it increases. Medical law after a while begins to consider the *heterogeneity of the subjects of this right* and the need for different types of people to preserve their 'specialness', which is expressed in a different understanding of the word 'health' and 'illness' for different types of people and different attitudes to medical technologies. For the present, it is very hard to imagine the differences in such a legal environment from what we see around us now.

What will be the consequences of the division of the medical legal environment on certain unequal areas to serve the needs of people with different structures and physiology of the body?

- First of all, the medical law will have to take into account the peculiarities of the birth of new individuals of the given type of people. These features can be very significant and moreover incompatible in people of different types. It may change the concepts of 'biological parents', 'pregnancy', 'prenatal period', 'accouchement', 'obstetric aid', 'twins', 'relative', and other familiar, self-evident concepts of today. Some concepts of the health law could become extinct. In return, there may appear fundamentally new rights: *the right of man to produce offspring of the selected type.*
- There may also appear a new human *right to live in an environment for which his body is adapted.* Thus, the right to choose their place of residence, which is now the subject of civil rights, can migrate to the medical law and become imperative along with the right to life and health. As a result, the concept of compensation for a need to temporarily stay in the environment to which the given organism is not adapted may appear.
- The right to medical care in the future may be integrated with the type of organism that receives such assistance. In

other words, to be eligible to provide medical assistance to a person with a certain type of body structure for the future health care workers, as well as for the clinics, one may need a separate medical licence. Equally, we can expect the patient's *right to obtain the assistance of a health professional in certain situations with the same type of structure of the organism as the patient has* to appear.

- In addition to the right to renounce the use of some medical technology for moral or religious reasons, the right to renounce the use of medical technology because of the danger changing the type of the patient's organism appears. In other words, the *right to save the the type of structure chosen by patient and functioning of his organism during the treatment* appears.
- *The concept of disability also may change.* In particular, the same medical condition, which arose spontaneously or as a result of therapeutic manipulation may be treated differently for different types of human organisms. For one type of body structure, it would be considered as normal, for another as a severe disability with appropriate legal consequences.
- Features of the structure and physiology of the body can lead to *significant changes in the other sections of civil law*, such as change in the age of legal capacity (majority), change in the age of consent, a change in the retirement age, and some others. The legislation will have the whole tables for calculating the age limits for certain legal entities with different types of organisms.

The definition of medical technology given in Section 2.C will need some clarification for now, as follows:

Medical technology is a combination of knowledge, skills, techniques, and equipment that enable a qualified specialist to affect the natural development and changes in biological objects *of given type* directly or indirectly, both individually and en masse, taking into account the reaction of the objects themselves and achieving goals with the greatest degree of probability. At a certain point, it becomes a tool for the health care systems *of appropriate types.*

That is, after a little while, to speak of medical technology 'in general' or about the health care system 'in general' would be impossible. We have to specify about what type of customers are referred to in this case. Change in the type of the organism of the HCS client, for example, as a result of some medical procedures, will lead to a radical change in the relations into which he enters into the health sector, as he will automatically go to the jurisdiction of other legislation (very similar to the current situation with the achievement of a man the age of majority, but even more radical) and become the client of HCS, based on entirely different principles. As soon as the various branches of humanity will specialise and adapt to different habitats, as well as the appearance and disappearance of these very artificial habitats, the move in the moral imperatives of these groups, in terms of the 'permissible' and 'unacceptable', as well as in the religious consciousness of these groups will inevitably occur. With the passage of time, a completely *separate type of medical care,* and, respectively, special health care systems based on them, designed for specific types of human organisms may appear.

Summary of the Fourth Chapter

Summing up the results of the fourth chapter, describing some scenarios for health care for the lifetime of the present generation of physicians (approximately up to 2050), it should be noted that these scenarios are a logical continuation of the processes that already started in medicine and health systems of most developed countries. It has been said that a person is most interested in a rather specific period of the future: the remaining years of his own life, plus lifespans of his children and grandchildren, which adds up to 150-200 years. Namely, this period we call 'future' in the everyday sense of the word. It is also said that the border of the future gradually moves away from us, and as life expectancy increases, humanity begins to call the 'future' period of 300 years or more.

The emergence of breakthrough technologies in medicine and public health can be expected:

1. The needs for satisfaction of which the new technology will be used should actually exist in the public consciousness, and awareness of this need should occur before a discovery or invention.
2. Practical application of the invention should not require new discoveries and inventions, i.e. be technologically implementable at the moment.
3. For the transition to the new technology, there should be ready-to-use science base; in particular, there should be ready tools for monitoring and measuring the results of the new technology.

The scenario of bionic prosthetics of lost limbs, organs, and their individual functions has been specified as one of the possible scenarios of a breakthrough medical technology. Over time, this technology may go on to create fundamentally new organs that would be needed for a person under certain circumstances, professional needs, or in special habitats. Also, it can be used to improve the communication capabilities of initially healthy people, creating new ways of socialisation of the population, the acquisition of new skills, the emergence of a fundamentally new jobs and new professions. Prosthetics can completely change the face of preventive medicine; in particular, it may be possible to change the properties of human organs and systems so that failures do not occur at all or would occur at a much later age. It may also be possible to protect the organs and their separate functions in advance from injuries and damages for some profession or age groups.

A question was raised about the danger of turning the patient's body into an object of patent protection because of the mass of bionic devices inside his body and also because of the possible aesthetic and artistic manipulations of his appearance. It was pointed out that the ways out of this situation are only two: either create a government's financial structure, which would carry out all the payments to the owners of patents on behalf of prosthetic citizens, or to limit the patent law itself, completely eliminating from it all the biological objects. Both decisions will be advantageous and disadvantageous.

Further, it was predicted that in the near future the state of *all its citizens will be considered as patients*, by definition. In such circumstances, the state no longer needs the formal permission from a person for diagnostic activity. This transition is the most important change in the paradigm of actions of the medical person from the earliest times. In this case, HCS is gradually moving towards the concept of continuous monitoring of the patients, i.e. all its citizens. Namely, this concept can realise the dream of preventive medicine that can not be reliably implemented under conditions of technological stage of external subjective or instrumental medical examinations. There will be a gradual transition to the creation of a universal friendly living environment, which keeps track of all members of the species Homo sapiens that are living inside. This habitat is a completely new tool for collecting data on the human population in general.

In the pharmaceutical industry, a *gradual abandonment of the concept of mass production of finished products 'for all' in favour of the concept of the production of personalised medicines for narrow target groups of patients*, as well as the production of 'pharmaceutical intermediates', designed to rework in specialised pharmacies will happen. The scheme of relations between the physician and the pharmacist can get back to a medieval version, when a doctor writes a prescription for the pharmacist who would prepare the individual drug for the individual patient. Questions of legal responsibility for treatment failure will be very inconvenient for practical use; they will have to subpoena a few dozen experts immediately. Inevitably, the entire treatment process will need to be broken down into individual technological stages that are available for reliable quality control and assign responsible professionals for each stage.

It has been said that the technologies of bionic prosthetics of individual organs and tissues, as well as the technology of growing the individual organs, can be developed. If this technology is implemented, then at some point it may be worth less than the traditional treatment of the patient. In this case, the treatment technologies will be very quickly, within a generation of doctors, left as economically inefficient and will be replaced by technologies of driven regeneration of organs.

As technology of bionic prosthetic organs and their individual features, people will already be born as adapted and specially designed for their living environment. What exactly are these living environments we cannot know in advance; it will be solved by the residents themselves: It is possible that originally the difference in air pressure, atmospheric composition, temperature and humidity, different kinds of radiation, etc. will be discussed.

It was concluded that humanity is becoming more *diverse* in terms of health. It conducts to the situation when the percentage of the population that can be officially recognised as healthy all the time is reduced, which gives the population a clear but false impression that the doctors and the health system as a whole are getting worse and worse to cope with their work. Thus, it will proceed to the artificial diversity of the human population, which will mark a new stage in its evolutionary development. Unlike earlier, this stage will be completely man-made. At some stage, there will appear the *different types of human organisms.*

It has been said that namely the work of the state to find a balance between all the participants in health and social processes leads to a fundamentally new branch of law, which was not in the classical Roman law, nor in the Civil Code of *Napoleon.* This section describes the *rules by which the given society reached agreement to control its quantity, longevity, and level of health.* The human society in its history did not experience such needs before. Changes in this legislation can lead to a completely separate type of medical care, and, accordingly, based on them are the separate health systems designed for specific types of human organisms.

Chapter 5

Scenarios of Medical Technology till 2100

The philosophies of one age have become the absurdities
of the next, and the foolishness of yesterday has become
the wisdom of tomorrow.

(Sir William Osler, 1849-1919)

In this section, I propose to try to predict the development of
medical technology, the rudiments of which do not exist yet and
which the current generation of doctors are likely to have no
chances to see. It is not so much about technologies of treatment
of diseases (at that time diseases will be an annoying minor
episode in the patient's life, which would have gone out of
the friendly living environment), but about the technologies of
improvement and transformation of organisms of all people, who
are patients by definition, about technologies that make the human
body characteristics and features, which biological evolution could
not have given him in principle, but which can give the artificial
techno-biological evolution. Can we call such the technologies as
medical yet?

5. A. Transplantation Endocrinology

After the discovery of hormones in the early twentieth century and their impact on the human body, the public and the scientific world were filled with high hopes for a quick victory over the majority of diseases. They also expressed hopes on decisive transformation of the human body through the manipulation of the endocrine glands. Eugenics got a second wind. Science-fiction writers of that time wrote works in which the human body changed as a plastic mass according to the desire of the endocrinologist. However, the degree of control, which they wanted to have, were not achieved because of many reasons.

I think that the reason for the failure was a lack of understanding of management principles, which governed the endocrine system of the body, as well as the inability to understand what the endocrine system is such, exactly where it begins and where it ends. Initially, it was thought that all hormones are specialised, and to manage the target organs, it is possible simply by entering the appropriate dose of required hormones. Only at the end of the twentieth century it was realised that the nervous, endocrine, and immune systems of the body were a single entity from the information point of view. And attempts to regulate the functions of the body by administering doses of specific hormones from the outside looked like an attempt to improve the video of the TV set by introducing the metal screwdriver in the rear panel—the result could be anything.

Endocrinologists of today are not trying to interfere with the processes of global governance of organs and systems but have more modest goals—treatment of insufficient or excessive functions of the endocrine glands. Today we know that endocrine cells are present in any organ and in almost every tissue of the human body and are ready when commanded to produce a huge range of hormones and their chemical precursors, thus performing 'ad hoc' current tasks for changing the functional state of the tissues in which they are located. All three of the managing systems: nervous, immune, and endocrine, are aimed at maintaining homeostasis. The nervous system is doing this at the behavioural level, the immune system at a structural, and the endocrine system at the functional level. All three systems interact with each other without involving the human mind to perform such constant and routine tasks. In the near future, the paradoxical medical task may appear: how to get all three systems that maintain the homeostasis not to oppose the doctors' efforts to change the human body as needed? The first to come across in such sort of tasks were transplantologists while attempting to 'negotiate' with the immune system so that it continued to work fine, but did not touch the transplanted organ. Without a solution of this problem in one form or another, the moving to a managed human evolution will be difficult; more precisely, it will be impossible.

In the future, endocrinologists will have to solve the issues of interaction between organs and tissues of the body in the same way as today's programmers solve the problems of integration between different software products using special rules for the information exchange—data transfer protocols. The job of IT-developers today is facilitated by the fact that all the protocols are described in the detailed specifications created by humans and obey certain logic. In addition, the programmer is sure that the programmes are not sharing information behind him by using a fundamentally different way of communication and that this mode of communication is not available to his senses and his understanding. A modern endocrinologist is extremely limited in its ability; through today's clinical and instrumental methods, he sees only a very small part of the information exchanged between the organs and body systems. Making the medical decisions based on such scant and fragmentary information is extremely dangerous, and this risk has been understood since the dawn of endocrinology. Problem is that endocrinology itself a science, because of the limitations of its methods, cannot capture the whole picture of information exchange between the organs and tissues in the body and therefore is not able to intervene in a meaningful way for the correction of the information entity which our body is. In the near future, we can predict the merger of several medical specialties: endocrinology, neurology, cytology, immunology, and medical genetics, in a supra-specialty concerned with the issue of internal control of terrestrial organisms in general and, in particular, the human body, as well as issues of information exchange between organisms. Currently, I propose to call this future science as *bio-cybernetics*, but in that, the part of it, which will cover the human body, will be *medical bio-cybernetics*.

In terms of such a science, all organs and tissues of the human body will be informational entities that receive the specific signals from the environment and from each other and change their functional status on the basis of received information (not forgetting to notify the control centre). I agree that it is very similar to how the current system's engineers and integrators install and re-install software on servers that form a network. If necessary to arrange a fundamentally new service for users of this network, they just write a new programme that is perfect for their purpose and uses the same transmission protocol; otherwise this program will be a foreign body for the system. Future biocybernetics will be able to read any information shared between organs and systems, regardless of how (which protocol) it's transmitted: nervous, humoral, or by modifying and encoding the specific proteins on cell membranes. I'm sure that other ways to transfer data within cells, within tissues, within the body, and within the community of organisms (population) will be discovered. We do not know yet how to detect these signals, but it does not mean that they do not exist. All this diversity of information exchange is the inheritance of the multibillion history of life on Earth; they emerged in different periods of the planet, when the basic conditions of life were fundamentally different, so it is not surprising to see the diversity of ways in which this biological information is transmitted. It can be said that these protocols were adopted by organisms at different times, in different geological and climatic eras; moreover, the nature of the transmitted information was different, just as different was the definition of the organism in those times. Superposition of multiple data protocols on top of another is a logical result of evolution, which has experienced several planetary biological disasters, after which the surviving organisms had to re-produce the rules of information exchange.

Knowing the full picture of information exchange in the body at one level, for example, on the interstitial level, future biocybernetics can meaningfully intervene in the management of the body, knowing exactly what he is doing and what will be the consequences of this intervention at the macro level. Clearly, the commands must meet the way of data passing; some of the commands can be transmitted only through hormones, and some can be transmitted only through the nerve synapses. All these messages are transmitted at very different speeds and in addition also have a different priority in the system. All these difficulties should not frighten us, because all this we can observe in the modern networking technology and telecommunications, and already it is clear that all of these problems are solvable.

Similarly, as a modern programmer does not enter manually the bytes for management of information system into the channels of communication, but writes specialised programmes which humans with inaccessible speed are able to assess the situation and, according to the developed algorithm, can correct it, the future biocybernetists cannot just enter the individual control signals to the system, but entrusts it to the specially designed information entities: biocybernetical artificial organs. These control centres may look like artificial endocrine glands, artificial nerve centres, and pools of cells with specific membrane proteins, which are able to change its configuration. These control centres will be recognised by the body as its own, because they will use the same communication protocol as the natural tissues. But they will have a significant difference: They will obey external commands of human, given by a high-level language. From a programmer's perspective, the control centre will be the interface that is the way of translation (encoding) information received from a doctor in its own codes of the body. It is very important that this interface can send commands with the usual body speed and frequency, even in the absence of a doctor.

Manipulation of the functional states of human organs and tissues can provide multiple effects that address both medical and non-medical problems, such as the following:

- They make human organs and tissues that are exposed to microbial attack and the simplest as completely unsuitable for their functioning, which can free the humanity from the whole classes of infectious and parasitic diseases, as well as from helminthiasis. This single change could save billions of dollars in funds that are spent on the production of antibiotics and vaccines and save millions of lives.

- Stimulating the production of additional haemoglobin, it's possible to make mankind live and work in high mountains that will give immediate benefits to the appropriate countries and territories. The same change can dramatically improve athletic performance in any sport, and for all newcomers. In medical terms, this can greatly facilitate the course of the diseases associated with ischemic damage to organs and tissues, as well as to exclude certain types of anaemia.

- Causing the human hepatocytes to produce specific antidotes, the mortality from poisoning by some specific natural poisons and industrial waste can be dramatically reduced, as well as significantly easier for diseases associated with toxicosis, including pregnancy. Diabetes can completely escape into the past by mastering the art to create and maintain the population of insulin-producing cells in all tissues of the patient.

- By changing the functional state of human adipose tissue finally, it will be possible to solve the global problem of weight loss. Everyone will have the shape and weight of body that is comfortable for him in the moment and will change it according to changing the life circumstances.
- By slightly changing the composition and acidity of saliva produced by our salivary glands, you can completely change the and perhaps almost destroy the flora in our mouth that will give a huge economic effect: Humanity altogether ceases to suffer from tooth decay, thus, will save hundreds of billions for treatment and prevention of such. Specialty 'dentists' will be much more rare than they are now.
- By suppressing vital functions of hair follicles, you can dramatically slow the growth of hair on the head, which will annually save on the national economy at the hairdressers. Further economic effect can enable the opportunity to artificially slow down or even stop the growth of hair on the face and body. We cannot even imagine the number of man hours that we spend on daily on shaving, as well as the production and purchase of shaving and hair removal products. The time and money can and should find a much more useful application.

These seemingly small changes in the functional state of organs and tissues in the mass can so dramatically change the daily life and the economy of mankind that today we cannot estimate the value of these improvements. The release of huge economic resources are now employing unproductive activities that serve the needs caused by some features of the human body and can completely change the planetary economy, freeing up billions of man hours for more creative work. There will come a time to realise that these features of the structure and physiology are given to us by inheritance from very distant ancestors (some even from simple organisms), and we absolutely do not need them more in an artificial environment in which our species lived for centuries.

In the next chapter, we will see how can another control system of our body be changed—the nervous system, and what are the consequences that this may cause.

5. B. Neuro-Programming and Simulation: Copyright on Thoughts and Emotions

The ancient anatomists were at a loss when trying to understand the purpose of the organ located in the skull of mammals and humans. The most annoying was the fact that scientists could not figure out what produces such a large gland and where is its secretion. A serious study of the brain function began only in the nineteenth century.

Now we know what we wear on our shoulders is a complex electrochemical analog computer for storage of prepared solutions and strategies of behaviour for all cases that may arise in the life of a particular representative of the species, as well as for developing new solutions of problems that is not provided by the vital programme of the given species. Recently, the main efforts of neuroscientists focused on understanding how to encode the information used by the nervous system while collecting the data from the peripheral organs, its processing, and returning to the lower level to respond to the problem. There have been some advances in the understanding of motor commands arising in certain areas of the brain, which give great hope for the development of a reliable human-machine interface that allows you to translate 'desire' of a particular person in the computer code to perform the required movements of mechanical devices. Experimental developments in this area are ready for commercial use.

With the inverse problem of creating a machine-human interface, things are much worse, because giving the digital commands into the electrochemical analog computing device of an unknown design is a rather intricate task. It's still too early to go into details of the technology, and it makes little sense: It is not the subject of this book. It is much more interesting to try to predict how the world will change after the creation of reliable communication systems between man-made and natural analog devices that allow computers to communicate with our brain and how this will change humans as a species.

The first thing that will be done, by the logic of human nature, is the creation of the stock of knowledge, facts, and skills, which the brain could load if necessary for a fuller picture of the world. That is, it is about a 'hard drive', which would be able to read directly from the brain or at least by its periphery—the organs of senses. Actually, the introduction of information to the brain from external media had been used by mankind long ago: books that are perceived through sight. The situation will be changed dramatically just with the super-fast reading of information that could be even more or less comparable to the reading speed of hard drives of computers. This technology will revolutionise the process of education and vocational training and retraining, saving the millions of man hours on the creative and intellectual labour. It'll change the very purpose of education of children, who in the presence of this technology will become adults much faster. This technology will be a prototype of the *next human signalling system*: ultra-fast transfer of knowledge from brain to brain via a mediator; thus the most important function of the brain as a place to store the facts and winning strategies of behaviour for the first time in the history of mankind become external and, moreover, amenable to centralised and mass modifications.

We cannot even imagine now fully the consequences of such an improvement but rather add-ins of our nervous system. Imagine a world in which every single fact or information that will need your brain for making some conclusions or calculations appears 'on demand' in a matter of seconds, but the human mind does not even register the fact that the external data source was used. A person will feel that he 'remembered' the required data. In such circumstances, the scientific activities will also be completely transformed: The most difficult part of any study (search and comparison of data in the literature) will take place within the brain of the researcher; at that time, the results of such activity will be ready-made conclusions about the suitability of the given data for the study of this phenomenon.

If the ready-made facts could be transferred in the brain, the next logical step would be inevitable: introduction of the techniques into the brain, allowing one to make the right conclusions and generalisations of the provided information, its structuring; that is, they will proceed to a partially programmable brain activity. A person using such software will be far above his contemporaries in their thinking abilities just as the great thinkers of the Enlightenment and Renaissance periods were above the provincial poor peasants in France or Spain. Clearly, all these sets of ready facts and techniques for finding and structuring information are not something entirely new in the history, because namely the 'filling in' of this content in the brain is the essence of teaching children and adults in the present time. The principal difference will be with very low laboriousness and at a very high speed of learning theory and practical skills, as well as full control over the quantity and quality of information 'loaded' into the brain with such technology. Super-fast technology of 'loading' information into the human brain will radically change the situation with the transmission of collected information to the future generations and will affect the species of Homo sapiens as a whole:

- It can by an order of magnitude increase the speed of learning for both children and adults. Herewith, the theoretical and practical vocational training of children can begin much earlier, given that the future professions will no longer require considerable physical efforts. The high rate of entry of new individuals into adulthood is an important strategic factor in the survival of any species.
- Humanity will be able to conduct a very flexible policy in professional employment, because with that speed of training a person can try dozens of different professions in his life and make significant progress in each. Professional

skills of several specialties will be superimposed on each other for life; that will give a new quality: everyone will know and be able to do 'almost all'; the boundaries of professions will blur, and it will difficult to say in which area the given person works.

- Nothing will prevent the organising of news channels on various topics in the future, information from which will go directly to the brain of the consumer at his request. The appropriate target audience of humanity will be informed about current events almost instantaneously and simultaneously. There will be a sharp increase in the volume and the rate of arrival in the latest scientific information.

- The vocational training of specialists can go to the next level: With the introduction of the appropriate information into the brain of trainee, you can simulate the occurrence of certain learning situations and check the resulting reactions and ways of handling these situations in his mind. This is similar to automated software testing. The examinee cannot distinguish between simulation of a learning situation and its actual occurrence; thus, the monitoring of the effectiveness of the theoretical and practical training is increased by an order.

- At some stage, the information that enters the brain may be subject to copyright; in particular, it may be the methods and algorithms for processing of data. The copyright on specific methods of information processing in the brain is practically very difficult to distinguish from the copyright on ideas that occur during data processing.

Note that we only discuss the consequences of the implementation of the method of superfast downloading of the information into the brain of the consumer. The reverse process— reading the analog data that are stored in the brain (including the contents of long-term memory) and writing it down into the medium—is not even discussed yet.

Another big change in the lives of people can relate to discovering a method of control of subconscious brain activity. It is about the content of our long-term memory, which, in essence, makes us unique individual personalities. If they will discover a way to write down into the person's memories events that did not occur with him in reality (false memory), it will forever change our personalities, largely virtualising them. And then the phrase posed in the title will begin to make sense. The new signalling system of humans, which is a data exchange system, methods of processing, as well as recording the sequences of emotions directly from the brain to the brain, will inevitably lead to the emergence of a new law section: *copyright on the thoughts and emotions in the mind of another person*. Many authors acknowledge that information is becoming the most important goods and services which humanity produces, and this will inevitably entail the legal consequences. Now we cannot even imagine how this can be technically arranged, but the rights to consuming of data, thoughts, and emotions of others will be earned.

Add-ins of the human nervous system are not just the improvement that may affect our species. The next step is improving all the functions of our body, as well as the fashion of the structure of the body, but we'll learn more about this in the next chapter.

5. C. Body Engineering: Human As an Art Object.

Since time immemorial, people tried to decorate their body. The need for clothing is irrelevant in this case, although the design of clothing is an important element of designing oneself as an art object. Even those tribes who live in equatorial Africa and throughout the year do not need clothes decorate their bodies in various ways. Archaeologists, excavating the burial sites of Stone or Bronze Age, can see only the skeleton of the hero of the day and the remains of its stone and metal jewellery; they are not able to see how people really looked at the time. I think if they could see them, they would be greatly surprised.

The view about their own beauty in the representatives of all human races has deep innate biological grounds. Polish anthropologist Ludwig Krzhivitsky in the book *Anthropology* said, 'Each group considers itself the most beautiful, until they meet up with other, more powerful. Tasmanians looked at their black color, as the pearl of perfection, and advised Europeans be smeared with charcoal in order to hide his ugliness that is white skin.' Austria's best specialist in the field of ethology Konrad Lorenz wrote: 'Our aesthetic perception is clearly related to the bodily changes.' A hundred years before, the best anthropologist Frenchman Paul Topinar adhered to similar beliefs: 'People with round heads argue that this form is most sublime. The Chinese claim that the flat face and slanting eyes are the pearl creation. According to the Negro, the most beautiful color is black.' Thus, the values of criteria of perception among people of different races are derivatives of the functions of the structure of their body. For example, the Chinese people, and in general all the people of the Mongoloid race, naturally have small feet, but the women of the upper classes sought artificial means to make the girls' legs even smaller. Tahitians, gottentony, and many island nations considered a wide, flat nose particularly beautiful, which was peculiar to them, and not surprisingly, they tried to flatten noses and foreheads of their children to make them more flat and attractive. Many peoples flattened the skulls of their children; it is obvious that they did so for the most part from a desire to give shape to their skulls, which was observed only in distinguished persons.

There is a tendency to mutilation or alteration of the natural shape of some body parts inherent to human nature at all levels as the most primitive and barbaric and the most civilised and spiritual, continuously reproducing generation after generation. This tendency is perpetuated with imitation, which, according to Herbert Spencer, may stem from two divergent reasons: either out of respect for the one who is mimicked or the desire to catch up with him. The quest for artificial deformations of the body in representatives of some ethnic groups is associated with their awareness of their own imperfections of structure. Namely, a subjective feeling of inherent physical inferiority makes them perform these 'modifications' of natural condition.

The crude form of tattoo art is practiced by already extinct Tasmanians and certain tribes of Australians, on the naked bodies of whom you can see straight or convex oval scars arranged in a certain way on the shoulders and chests. Tattoos may substantially mitigate or even completely destroy the impression of nudity in these nations. Often mothers tattooed their children to identify them by the tattoos, if they were abducted afterwards. Tattoos have served also as talismans and distinctive signs, signs of health, and puberty; also, they pointed to the marital status. In ancient Japan, a man with a tattoo who was a persona non grata was banished from society and family and condemned to complete isolation. Tattoos were usually made in a conspicuous place on the bodies of criminals, and they could even tell in which prison they were serving sentences. The base of painting and tattooing is purely decorative now, but thick scars of different types can already be seen as a transitional step to artificial changes of body shape. The first place among these changes belongs to changing the shape of the skull, which included trying to detach the child's head in early childhood with special tools or bandages. The custom of artificial changing of the shape of the head is one of the oldest and most widely known customs, which is found under various modifications in various parts of the world among people who do not communicate with each other.

This long introduction was given to prove a simple fact that all the tools available to them at the moment are used by people to change their body and appearance as it seems beautiful at the moment, and this happens in all people, as they say, 'without saying a word'. The key statement here, I think, is the phrase 'tools available to him at the moment'. Progress in the field of biomedical technology, bionics, and microelectronics is moving at a pace that in the near future people will get the tools to enable them to not only decorate their body, as did our ancestors, but also overbuild on it and alter it. The rate of change in the concept of 'beautiful' is already so high that fashion in clothes and appearance changes every few years, and these trends are becoming more and more man-made. Earlier, fashion for exterior appearances in the ancient world continued for centuries; in the Middle Ages, it was for decades, but now, a change occurs every two to three years. It is logical to assume that in a few decades the concept of 'beautiful' for different groups of mankind will change several times a year. The amount of resources consumed to meet this human need is growing like an avalanche. Even now the amount of funds, which is spent on cosmetics, body care, fashion, plastic surgery of different scales, and fitness in developed countries, exceed the defence budgets of these countries.

So far, people are not changing their bodies just because they know that reversing these changes will not be possible. Most people who want to make a tattoo do not do it just because it will be almost impossible to remove it. People generally do not like to do irreversible steps. As soon as the technology will reversibly change the human body, there will be an *explosion in the consumer market of body alterations.* Humanity should be rational in thinking about the shortcomings and dangers of these technologies and foreseeing some legal restrictions in this area. For example, it would be rational to consider the following:

- Despite the alterations of person's body, the *indestructible sign by which he can be quickly and reliably distinguished from other members of the species* should remain. Once it was the appearance, then it was the name in document, the fingerprints, but now it is the picture of the iris. What will be the identification sign of a personality in a world where any part of the human body can be changed?
- *Limit size of the body, both upward and downward.* This is particularly important for use by a specific person, most of the benefits which are important to civilisation: transportation, shelter, access to information, safety devices. Imagine a man who grows his body to rise above 3 metres and a weight of 300 kg. Do you think he will be able to use all the planes, trains, elevators, live in a hotel or a train compartment, be treated in the hospital, or use the standard means of salvation in case of fire?
- *Alterations of the body that are changing or eliminating the reproduction function of the individual.* In fact, if society would allow people to eliminate en masse (for any reason) their ability to reproduce, will it affect the quantity of the human species, especially if it happens before the discovery of the method of in vitro reproduction? Should the legislation ban or restrict this practice, especially when we consider that it is practiced already in some countries?
- *Alterations of the human body that would prevent normal operation of automatic safety systems in public places or in transport.* In particular, it includes alterations that deliberately disorient such systems while recognising a person or causing a false report about the danger.

- *Alterations of the body and the nervous system* which somehow or the other are *preventing child's learning.*
- *Alterations of the body, affecting the definition of the biological age of the individual.* In fact, the danger of such massive alterations to hide age is underestimated. Imagine a society where it is fashionable to look under twenty-five years, and *all* of the adults rework their bodies so that they become even instrumentally indistinguishable from the twenty-five-year-old. A huge number of aspects of our life are organised around our knowledge of the date of birth. In the case of deliberate concealment of this parameter, many sides of the organisation of human life may be virtually locked: education, career development and employment law, serving in the army and security units, the onset of age of legal capacity and age to marriage, voting rights, health care, and insurance (also including medical).

Such limitations will be necessarily agreed in advance, 'on the bank', because the people whose bodies were changed 'against the rules' will fall into the legal trap, and after the adoption of laws, they will be out of the society for rest of their lives. Cannot be excluded the appearance of a new section of the legislation, which would describe the right of citizens to change their bodies as well as the bodies of their minor children. This section of law will govern the relationship between people with different structures and features of the bodies, with physical limitations, and vice versa, with new physical and psychological capabilities. Equally, it will adjust some of the limitations which people will not overcome while they change and improve their organisms, including the punishment of infractions of these rules.

The human body may well be the bearer of a new art form, the name of which has not yet been derived. The modern term 'body art' absolutely cannot describe the opportunities that will become available to mankind in the design of their bodies. We are concerned not only about the external features of the body, the cosmetic changes that are already on the verge of art, which we call 'make-up', but also namely about the design of the functional content of the human body. New and enhanced features of the body can bring a completely new feel to the owners, making it possible to experience a new range of emotions that make up the content and value of any art. Opportunity to wear the art inside itself as an integral part of his body is a completely new feature for the humans. Until now, the art was always something external and required a certain instrument or carrier. Particularly acute experiences will give the possibility of changing the design of their body during life, like changing the tastes and needs of the individual. For the first time in human history, the body will become *temporary*.

All such changes and superstructures of the body, as well as the nervous system, will lead to a lengthening of the human life, which will cause changes in the mentality of the average man, his attitude towards himself, his health, and his offspring. Along with the increase in the lifespan, the changes in the economy of mankind, which is tied to the average duration of the human life, are much more than what people think.

5. D. Social and Health Care Consequences of Practical Immortality

Despite the fact that the title sounds absolutely fantastic, consideration of that can help us to make far-reaching practical conclusions and to understand, first of all, if the idea of immortality is so good as mankind thinks. In the legends and myths of almost all nations, there are some creatures that live if not forever then very long in comparison with ordinary people. Such beings were deified, as such a long life has always been considered an attribute of the divine, non-human origin. Longevity was considered a gift of the gods long before the appearance of health systems, which set the goal of human life longevity on an industrial base.

To understand the impact of the significant lengthening of human life it is not necessarily predicted in detail how namely this can be done. Details of the technology are not important here, but the result is important, just like for the discussion of the impact of transport problems it is not necessary to know the details of the design of engine installed on the means of transport. Instead of this, it is important to know the results which it achieves: load capacity, average speed of cargo, energy efficiency, ecological impact on the environment, and others. Which parameters of the achieved results are useful to know before trying to model the effects of technology that it dramatically lengthens the human life?

First of all, you must know *how much* the given hypothetical technology lengthens the human life. While the increase is relatively small, it is possible to measure the extra years, which an average member of the population receives. But when the increment in the lifespan becomes large and comparable to the natural duration of human life, consideration of some extra years becomes meaningless; the number of times should be counted, which increases the lifespan of the average member of the population in comparison with terms if this technology is not used. The easiest way is to use the *coefficient of elongation of human life.*

Also an important indicator is the *selectivity* of technology, that is, the percentage of members of the population that can receive the coefficient of the elongation of life, mentioned in the preceding paragraph. They have to introduce another factor to characterise the selectivity of technology. If the technology will be applicable to any human being, the coefficient will be equal to 1, if only to the half of the population—0.5.

An important indicator could be also the *minimum age of using technology*; that is, is it possible to apply it to the newborn (and perhaps even to the foetus), or will the person need to live up to a certain age so this hypothetical technology can be effectively applied? The existence of such an indicator will automatically mean that the life of any person will be divided into two parts: before the application of life's extension technology and after that.

Another important parameter is *the ability to dosage*. In other words, will it be possible to extend the life of people several times for the pre-determined number of years, or a single application of the technology is only possible, according to the principle 'apply and forget'? This parameter will give citizens the possibility accurately enough to plan the duration of their lives and increase the availability of technology for people because of the lower price.

It will be one more feature of technology, the type of prolonging life. Logically I see three types of life extension: *Type 1*—the prolongation of life on the basis of 'stopping the ageing processes', *Type 2*—the prolongation of life on the basis of 'stopping the development of chronic diseases, including cancer', and *Type 3*—'replacing the failed organs with bionic prostheses and cyber-organic units'. They all give a significant (in times) prolongation of life, but life will be of different qualities. I will try to consider below what will be these qualities.

All of the above parameters will be merged; thus, all together they will determine the most important factor—*psychological changes*, in patients after implementation of this technology, resulting in completely different life motivations of these people, changing their attitudes towards themselves, their and other people's health, their own offspring, and their relation to health care system and its financing. Namely, changing the people's attitudes to themselves is the most important consequence of the rapid lengthening of human life in general.

The discovery of such a technology will trigger a snowslip of economic and demographic consequences, enabling the lifetime of one generation to change the entire social and industrial life of humanity, and it must be remembered that such changes always lead to severe economic crises. Economic activity of mankind is very much tied to the average life of the current generations; any sudden change in these terms will lead to economic shocks.

Example 1: Let's imagine that tomorrow we will know about the existence of life-prolonging technology, which doubles the lifetime of 50% of population using the first type of prolongation ('stopping the ageing processes'). Let's accept it as a fact that if the initial life expectancy was equal to eighty years. What will be the social and health care consequences?

Attitude to technology at this point will be drastically different for people of different ages and incomes. The biggest beneficiaries will be the young and affluent patients (technology initially will be very expensive), because they will prolong their life beginning from their youth. If they apply this technology to twenty-five-year-old person, the gain will be of 55 years (average age of survival to 80) × 2 = 110 years. The total time of that person's life would be 110 + 25 = 135 years. For the elderly and wealthy person who are aged 60 the gain would be much less: 20 years × 2 = 40 years, with a total lifespan of 60 + 40 = 100. If the technology is applied to the newborn, his average lifetime will be: 80 × 2 = 160 years. Less affluent citizens, for which this technology will not be available, will continue to live an average of 80 years. It becomes clear that the man who knows in advance that he can live up to 160 years and the man who knows that his limit is 80 years will have different self-conscience and different planning of their lives.

With the increase in the numbers of people with an extended average lifespan the demographic consequences will increase. It would begin to accumulate the elderly population, and as a result of globalisation, it will be distributed in all areas, not just in developed countries, where the technology of life extension is applied. Thus, all countries, not just developed ones, will have to immediately begin a range of socio-economic arrangements to compensate for distortions in the demographic structure of society. What do they need to fear in the first place?

In developed countries, namely, the elderly will be the first for whom this technology will be used, because, firstly, they will have free money and, secondly, the rest of the age cohorts will think that they have more time to think and look at the implications of this technology for others. In other words, the elderly will have nowhere to retreat. As a result, the demographic pyramid in the shape of 'burial urns' will begin to expand at the level of older age cohorts. The bottom of the pyramid, represented by the working population, will become narrower and narrower as compared with its upper part. Thus, all the problems related to the lack of labour force will further intensify. The number of retirees will grow rapidly in all countries, not just in the leading economic ones, which will very quickly lead to total and simultaneous collapse of pension funds. This problem will lead to the fact that new retirees would lose money that they could spend on the extension of their life. As soon as new retirees will become poor, the population pyramid will gradually come to its natural form (see Section 3.C), and the percentage of elderly people in the society will cease to grow. This will be the end of a cycle, phase 5; the demographic transition would be complete. At the end of the cycle, the population pyramid for several decades will have hitherto an unprecedented form: On top of it will form a 'bubble', represented by the older people who had applied to themselves the life extension technology, but age cohorts that followed them will not have such an opportunity because of poverty, because all pension funds will have already been used up. The bubble eventually will detach from the top of pyramid and hang 'in the air'; thus, the pyramid will split into two parts. Age cohorts, who turned in this 'bubble', very quickly will go out of this life, because for their maintenance and treatment the society will not have enough money. Remember that this type of technology is 'stopping the ageing processes', and that does not mean these long-living people will cease to being sick.

The consequence of this economic disaster will be that restoration of pension funds in their original form in the world will be impossible: Each government of each country will know how the elderly people will spend retirement money and what will happen with the economy in this case. Thus, the spreading of commercial technology for simply extending the life expectancy merely will lead to the immediate *collapse of the pension systems in all countries* that have not previously taken special fencing measures. Health system, as a part of the social protection systems, will also be on the brink of survival because of the sharp increase in the percentage of older clients for which the system was not designed. Protective legal measures taken by governments will provide only a temporary effect, since they will not completely cut off the channels of mass penetration of people with prolonged life.

Example 2: Now let's try to imagine the implications of technology of the second type (the exclusion of chronic diseases), which is effective in 100% of the members of the population in terms of application—22-23 years (the age of the end of growth), and elongates ALE by 50%.

In this case, the lives of all people will be divided into two unequal parts: before and after the application of the technology of life extension. This automatically means that all people older than twenty-three years will be practically healthy, except for those who became disabled after an injury and acute diseases. The old people will have the common involutional processes in the body, but they will not lead to chronic diseases. That is, the scourges of old age: hypertension, osteoarthritis, osteoporosis, atherosclerosis, vascular insufficiency, will not develop. In the past, this sometimes happened when the old man lived to a very old age and was never sick; it was said about him that he 'died of old age.' After application of the above technology of life extension, such an end of life can become universal. Note that the children and young people will continue to get sick from chronic diseases. What will be the social and health care consequences?

Let's calculate the new terms of life: $22 + (58 \times 1.5) = 109$. That is, all people will be able to live to about 110 years. It would seem that a great result would provide a general healthy ageing. Is it not for such a result that modern medical science is struggling? However, on closer examination, the situation is not so good.

The fact is that after a generation the healthy elderly people will nowhere be there to take in the presence of unhealthy children and adolescents. In fact, if a person in childhood has had all the childhood infections and gets the complication and while growing up gets a chronic disease, then in the age of 22-23 years, when undergoing technology for extending life, since he would have been originally sick, he will not get a significant advantage in terms of life. The entire health care system in such a society will be reduced and limited to only emergency care, paediatrics, and adolescent medicine. All the medical resources of society will be used to treat the children with only one goal—to keep any born child till they reach the age of using the life extension technology, with each new generation increasingly getting an unhealthy adult population. The more the greenhouse conditions will be created for children, the weaker the adults they will become. Weak adults will give birth to weaker children. This vicious circle will result in a drastic reduction of the population in a few generations. The population pyramid will become a 'pillar' of nearly equal width throughout, which slowly but surely will become narrower and narrower with each new generation. Under these circumstances, the existence of population will only be supported by sophisticated efforts of paediatricians. The number of working-age population after an initial period of growth will begin to taper off.

It becomes clear that with such technology of extending life it will be impossible to obtain the significant extended life, provided the technology allows us to use it from early childhood or even in the embryonic stage. Pension funds will have a chance to survive; the health system will survive, but will have a strong bias in favour of paediatrics and the treatment of trauma and emergency conditions.

Example 3: Finally, let's try to imagine the social and health consequences using the life extension technology of type 3—'replacing the failed organs with bionic prostheses and cyber-organic units' provided that it can be applied to a man from the embryonic stage and can be applied to the 100% of population with a coefficient of elongation of human life that is equal to 3. What is more, people will get the coefficient of 3 after replacing all his organs with prostheses.

Let's calculate the new average life expectancy: $80 \times 3 = 240$ years, and this duration of life will be for all those who are able to pay for replacement of all their failed organs with cyber-bionic nodes. For those who are born healthy and do not need of such changes, the terms of life remain the same and equal to 80 years. Mankind falls into a psychological trap: For prolonging their lives, people will try to replace even the healthy organs and will do this in the earliest ages to get more advantages for his lifespan. The time of replacement of organs will depend on the availability of funds to pay for such an operation. Thus, more affluent customers will replace their organs much earlier and will live much longer than the less wealthy. We can see how humanity is once again divided into two branches, only this time on the basis of the solvency. The separation process will be intensified because long-living (almost three times more) people will be, with each new generation, better educated and more intelligent than the short-living people. Labour productivity of them will be much higher. After several generations, the idea that somebody can live with the original natural organs would be unacceptable for the average person. Parents will not hesitate to apply the technology to their newborn children, trying to get the maximum long life for their offspring.

In such a society, the HCS in its curative side will be reduced to factories for production and storage of individual (customised) organs for people of all ages as well as hospitals for the installation, replacement, and maintenance of cyber-bionic prosthesis. From the medical specialties, the only familiar specialties will be obstetrics, which will look very different from what it is now, emergency care for injuries and poisoning, as well as some sections of medicine which control those diseases that cannot be cured by prosthetics.

5. E. New Occupations and Old Occupations: Everyone Treats Himself

If any of the early twentieth-century doctors would have heard the names of medical specialists that would be the most in demand in the early twenty-first century, they would not have even understand what exactly are these professionals; for them, it would be just words. In fact, words such as 'resuscitator', 'reflexologist', 'endocrinologist', 'microsurgeon', 'allergist', 'transfusiologist', and 'transplantologist' would not mean anything to them, because these sciences themselves did not exist yet. At the same time, old and familiar specialties, such as 'therapist', 'surgeon', 'obstetrician', and 'paediatrician', for 100 years have undergone tremendous changes in terms of content. Even the best therapist of the early twentieth century could not work in the modern clinic, despite the fact that the very subject of a professional application of knowledge does not change. Professional infrastructure has changed the content of specialties and the legislative field. What will happen with the health professions through the next 100 years? And how can we plan for it?

In fact, how can we prepare for the emergence of a new profession (even outside of medicine), if not only the methodological base for the preparation of such a professional but also the subject area is yet absent? Indeed, at the end of the nineteenth century, it would have not occurred to anyone create a flight school and build airfields before the invention of aircraft and cosmodromes before the creation of the first space rockets, despite the fact that the general idea of how these products will look like was already there. Any such infrastructure is built 'on the fact of' a specific technical invention and under its options. But in medicine this is not quite right; a new medical infrastructure is always created with new knowledge about the old object—the human body. *Organisationally the modern hospital was the direct successor of hospital in the late nineteenth century*; all of its functions, process steps and tasks of production, and, most importantly, the *philosophy* of industrial relations are largely preserved, as it deals with the same object of production. Teaching the new specialists in these conditions is much easier, because the basic knowledge in the specialties is almost unchanged. The first two or three courses of any medical college anywhere in the world (like a hundred years ago) is the study of the same anatomy, physiology, and general pathology.

If we trace the history of the medical knowledge of humanity in terms of a marketing relationship between physicians and patients, we have to admit that most of the history of this question will have to be described as a history of efforts for non-proliferation of such knowledge among non-physicians. Huge resources were spent on prevention of the spreading of the medical knowledge into the hands of patients. Here's how it is described by A. Toffler in his book *Powershift: Knowledge, Wealth and Violence at the Edge of the Twenty-first Century* (1990): 'For many years, doctors in the United States maintains an inaccessible power over medical knowledge. Recipes written on Latin, providing the profession, so to speak, semi-secret code that kept in the dark most of the patients. Medical journals and texts were addressed only to professional readers. Medical conferences were classified. Doctors monitored the curriculum and student admission to medical schools and universities.'

By the way, almost all the old professions that are more then 200 years old and associated with scientific knowledge have passed through this stage, from the navigator to the engineer and from the doctor to the theologian. They all passed the stage of corporate secrecy. In the twentieth century, there was a crisis: Widespread transition to universal secondary education has led to the impossibility of any further concealment and sacralisation of knowledge. Internet completes this process: *for now any professional (including medical) knowledge is available to everyone.* In such circumstances, how to protect the medical profession from the avalanche of non-professionals, who fragmentally read some facts about their illness and begin to start the treatment themselves, using the fact that the object of influence for this specialty is the exclusive property of each patient—their own bodies?

What happens to the professions when a new subject area appears? I propose to consider briefly the evolution of two new subject areas: aviation and automotive industry; firstly, they have appeared recently, just in the memory of the present generation, and secondly, they are absolutely new; that is, they do not have technology-progenitors.

For people, a job aviator in the late nineteenth century seemed a bit of a loony: a human smelling of kerosene, for days sitting in the shed (typically in a bicycle workshop, as in the case of the Wright brothers). He would design and assemble his aircraft. Then he would pilot it and repair it after an accident. Rare balloonists, who previously flew in the air in balloons, were not helpful in the design of machines heavier than air, which required complex technical skills and, most importantly, a different philosophy of flight. The same thing happened when the first cars came into existence; at first, no one counted them as the new mode of transport. They were considered just mechanical carriages, which were maintained and operated by steam engine mechanics, especially since the first models had steam engines. Thus, the first step in the development of a new profession is full of *universalism*: The whole cycle of works is performed by a single person, who has received his education on the new subject area of knowledge as a self-educated person. The feature of this phase is also the fact that the information concerning the new technology is not accessible to the public: Only the self-taught specialist understands the issues and has a direct interest in withholding information to save the market for its services. Is it not true that it is very similar to the ancient period of development of the medical profession?

Then it was possible to observe a very rapid decomposition of new professions on specialisation in relevant technological areas: designer, engineer, fitter, test pilot, operator, repairman, pilot, and navigator. This happened for two decades as in the aircraft industry and in the automotive industry. In medicine, this step took several centuries, and we cannot say that it's completely over. Why are processes of specialisation in medicine occurring so slowly, several times slower than in today's industry? I think it depends on the following factors:

- From the beginning, the object of professional application in medicine was not perceived as a technological object.
- The repair facility in medicine cannot be divided into process steps due to the inability to distinguish one problem from another. It was only in the late Middle Ages when scientists began to divide the human body into functional systems.
- There is immaturity in economic theory and management technologies that have evolved only in the middle of the nineteenth century. The emergence of cybernetics plays a significant role in the development of these technologies.
- The market of specialised medical services is narrow. The doctor who in the Middle Ages would have tried to specialise in, say, heart diseases (i.e. become a cardiologist) proved to be a pauper, because he could not separate the heart diseases from other problems. Those cases that clearly would have been cardiological could not suffice for his sustenance. In addition, the number of solvent patients in those days was so small that even a fully qualified modern cardiologist would just die of hunger.

Processes of specialisation in medicine are best monitored by the appearance of specialised departments at universities and medical schools; the first were the surgical and obstetric colleges. Later, they were separated also into other specialties: ophthalmologists, paediatricians, neurologists, and psychiatrists. Currently in universities, there are so many departments, each of which prepares physicians of narrow specialisation. There are authoritative opinions which are already sceptical that such narrow specialists in general can be called doctors. This is very similar to the situation when nobody would call 'aviator' a specialist of technical service for electronic systems providing the automatic landing of a modern airbus; thus, a new profession with a pretty clunky name was born. Did this expert regret that he could no longer build aircrafts and pilot them himself, as it was in the beginning of the twentieth century? I think that is unlikely. With the medical profession, the same thing happened, but we still cannot accept this. Universal doctors, as they were at the end of the eighteenth century, are no more and will not be. How far reaching is the specialisation of health professionals in the twenty-first century? Who can be called by the ancient word 'doctor' and can this profession remain as such?

Let's look at the profession 'motorist' and what has happened with it in the twentieth century.

Already in the 1920s, the profession began to divided by specialisations: *Garages* came into existence, i.e. specialised businesses in repair and maintenance of vehicles. Also, there came into existence the road services, networks of filling stations, and producers of fuel. In contrast, there appeared *chauffeurs*, whose work was to only control the vehicles. The very first cars were very expensive, and their owners who used the services of drivers could be counted on one hand. As cars were cheaper and cheaper, the number of private owners increased, and the owners themselves became 'chauffeurs'; that is, in the segment of personal cars the profession of *chauffeur* almost disappeared as early as the 1940s. Then there were citizens who could drive a car and those who could not. That is, the profession of 'driver' has become part of life skills of ordinary but advanced people on the Earth.

What's allowing some profession to be 'dissolved' among all the people? I think that this is necessary:

- Technology must be accessible to the ordinary citizen price wise.
- The technology must be easy to understand for an ordinary citizen; that is, he must understand on the whole 'how it works'. Or the average level of the education of citizens must rise to such a level that the technology would become clear to almost everyone.
- The technology must be simple and reliable to use; cases of failures and breakdowns should become quite rare.
- In order that the citizen should learn the profession and maintain his skills, the use of this technology should be frequent enough; that is, there should be the daily need for this technology. Use of a car is the daily need for now.
- The cost of failure of equipment should be low enough. The modern car breaks down fairly rarely, especially with professional care and timely replacement of spare parts. Thus, the price of failure is usually only the cost of replacing the broken parts. In aviation, the price of failure of equipment is very high—a fall with disastrous results; thus, this profession is very bad 'dissolving' among citizens, although by the price it is already available in many countries.
- Around the given profession, a specific infrastructure appears which allows citizens to learn the profession, obtain information about this technology, carry out the competent purchases in the market of this technology, repair and dispose off defective technical elements, and protect his rights, arising from his use of the technology.

All of these conditions have been met for the profession 'motorist'. The question posed in the title of the chapter is whether the profession *doctor* will go through all these stages. There is an avalanche of new specialisations in medicine, and around it, it grows. What it will end in terms of the organisation of the therapeutic process and to what extent the patient will be involved in this work?

If we look at the way how in the modern world the role of the patient has increased not only in the treatment of his own body but also in the formulation of the challenges faced by the health care providers in general, it becomes apparent that the number of functions delegated to the patient should move into quality. A patient with a higher education begins to understand not just the individual details of the medical technologies, not only to suggest the health professionals more rational ways of organising medical services for the community as a whole but also to articulate the common challenges facing the public health; that is, he begins to act like a normal customer at the macro level. Moreover, the automation of many routine medical procedures begins, thus, equipped and trained by physicians the patients themselves do such manipulations, which would be considered as absolute fantasy only 100 years ago. Now it seems ridiculous, but at the end of nineteenth century, the measuring of body temperature was considered as physician's manipulation. That is, the doctor with his own hands measures the patient's temperature. The patient did not have a thermometer at home; it was too complicated a device for him! Since then, a number of medical supplies and devices, which the patient uses in his own home, have been increasing. In particular, recently, the simple pregnancy tests that sold in every pharmacy made a revolution in obstetrics practice and which released the obstetricians from millions of unnecessary visits of patients who were interested in only one question. But for the entire mass of the same patients these cheapest tests saved billions in the national economy.

The *delegation* of certain powers to the client long ago began in non-medical fields of economy. In particular, many enterprises for repair of household appliances already advise their clients on the phone, figuring out the nature of the problem and recommending them what kind of simple repairs they should do. If necessary, they send a spare part by courier, or if this part is simple and often out of order, it is stored in the client's home! Only in really difficult cases will the professional be involved in repair. Thus, the repair process is intentionally divided into simple technological segments that are available for the understanding and implementation by the customer. In medicine, the same processes happen, but for the above reasons, they are much slower. In cases where they already can be implemented, as a pregnancy test, they give huge savings for the end user, which can be used to invest in the more professional approaches to the treatment and its organisation. What processes should we expect in health care management in the next 100 years?

As soon as medical specialisations will become more 'thinner' but the area of professional responsibility narrower, the opposite processes will start, namely, *the merger of several subspecialties into one*. For example, in my opinion, neurology, neurosurgery, and, oddly enough, ophthalmology and otology will have great chances to merge in the future. This assumption could be logical, if we remember that the eye and the inner ear are part of the brain, evolutionarily passed on to the periphery and specialised in the senses. That is, inverse merging of specialties may happen already not on the basis of treatment of a certain organ (as it was in the time of separation of specialties in the twentieth century) but on the principle of treatment of functional systems of the human body. Another platform for future integration of medical specialties is the treatment of clinical entities 'as a whole', at all of its stages, and regardless of the method of treatment. In future, health care policy-makers will be very surprised to hear that earlier the doctor who treated the ulcer conservatively, the doctor who treated the same ulcer surgically, and the doctor who was involved in its prevention were counted as doctors of various specialties, worked in different medical units, and competed with each other. In the world long ago there were small clinics that dealt with the prevention and treatment at different stages of a single nosological entity. The issue of sharing such a practice with all known nosological entities a matter of economics and law in the given country. The most important factor in this approach is the number of paying customers with this nosology and their mobility. Thus, the most common nosologies will the first to receive a highly specialised network of full cycle clinics.

The first step to be ensured that the medical profession is beginning to dissolve in the population is a rapid expansion of domestic medical and diagnostic devices. In particular, the spreading in the world of glucose meters, blood pressure monitors and heart rate monitors, electronic thermometers, portable equipment for physical therapy, instruments for electropuncture, and other equipment has led to the fact that more and more significant part of the diagnostic (and partly curative) activities are taking place at the home of the patient that is saving tens of thousands of man hours for medical staff and huge funds of patients. Now the patient goes to the doctor with a ready 'half stuff': a set of symptoms objectively proven by portable diagnostic devices. For the time being, these tools are very simple and give only one or a few parameters that the doctor has to verify in the clinic, but soon the hour will come when in a domestic environment a serious professional medical examination can be carried out. The question is the degree of power and miniaturisation of home diagnostic devices. Thus, some of the work of today's doctors—namely, diagnostic activity, is *leaving the doctor's hands and going into the hands of the client*. Public opinion is gradually moving to the concept that small repairs of his own body is the duty of the citizen and that the inability to do so is a sign of backwardness and lack of education. What would one now think about a young man who does not know how to replace the battery in a mobile phone or update the software in his media player and go for it in the corporate services?

Transition to the concept of 'medical self-service' of the population will require compliance with all the conditions that were listed above for the profession 'motorist', namely, the following:

- *Availability*: Simple diagnostic tools and technologies of small repair of his body will be available at the price of an ordinary citizen.
- *Understanding*: The average level of understanding of the citizen of the design of his own body will allow everybody to use automated diagnostic tools and understand the results they produce. It is possible that the basics of medicine will be a routine subject for secondary school.
- *Reliability*: It's not so much the issue of lack of equipment breakdowns as the reliability and validity of the results issued. Equally important is the inability to use this technique for other purposes or to harm each other.
- *The everyday need for technology*: So far the citizens do not perceive the need for everyday monitoring of the state of his body and the need for his current minor repairs. But, this situation will not last long. When a person's health will be a real factor in his ability to work, especially if in many professions the workability will evaluate the technique, the constant self-control of his health by monitoring some of the parameters and their correction will be an everyday habit and demand.
- *The low cost of failure*: Here we can talk about that the price of the diagnostic device errors as well as the price of the wrong actions by repair of the body should be as low as possible. It's hard to imagine the evolutional way how it would go, but one of such possible ways described in the

preceding chapters, which is the controlled regeneration of tissues and organs.

- *Infrastructure*: Specific infrastructure around the medical profession is already beginning to form—that there are NGOs of patients who teach their members self-diagnostics and first aid to each other and gives courses in first aid to the public and also specialised classes in high schools and colleges with intensive study of human anatomy and physiology and magazines for those interested in medical technologies and special news feeds in the field of medicine and more. In developed countries, there are public councils at major hospitals to enable the local community to participate in the management of the local hospital. This is a completely new phenomenon, which characterises the level of the population as a conscious customer of not only specific health services but also in the way of their organisation and payments.

These processes gradually lead to a situation where the *medical profession is 'dissolving' in the population*; that is, every able-bodied person would have the credentials to diagnose and treat a certain spectrum of diseases characterised by a low price of mistake. Just as it is now in most countries, the experienced mother does not call the doctor if her child has a cold, but quite successfully treats it with the contents of the home kit. Such credentials may coincide with the area of responsibility of a modern family doctor. In the case of more serious pathology, the given citizen will be cured by a pre-known medical specialist. Namely, these specialists will be called 'doctors' in the future, but the area of responsibility for most of them will not coincide with the modern specialisations. There will very different narrow medical specialties with new unfamiliar names; simultaneously, the familiar names of subspecialities will completely change their meaning and content.

Conclusions. Outlines of Future Health Care

So, reading the book is finished. We considered the development of medicine and public health at an angle at which it is very rarely seen even by the experts, and it must be said that this picture was perceived by modern man not without inner resistance. But that's OK. The lifestyle of descendants always seems deeply flawed and wrong for their ancestors. If somebody would have said to Europeans in eleventh to twelfth century that after 800 years half of Europeans would be atheists, they would have preferred to do all you wanted, just so that such a future would not come true, as that would have been nothing worse than they could imagine. Ability to consider the future from the standpoint of benefit for future generations is the art little mastered by man yet.

As you were reading the book, many familiar concepts from childhood have been redefined; in particular, the concept of medicine has been redefined:

> *Medicine* is a complex of knowledge and technologies based on them that allow the species to perform the selective breeding within its own species, having the purpose of countering the natural processes that inhibit the expansion of this species on the entire habitat available for him. It occurs at a certain stage of development of the species, when some of its individuals are able to affect the life expectancy and rate of reproduction in this and other species.

This new definition gives us an understanding of medicine as a social mechanism for artificial selection in the interests of a particular species, what is more, any sufficiently advanced species. In the first chapter, it was concluded that the conscious breeder that's performing the self-selection in human society is precisely the health care system, not individual doctors. The quality of health system is largely determined by the fact that the system itself 'understands' whom and why it chooses. It was also shown that a group of doctors, even the most skilled, is not yet the health care system; it becomes such when it understands its goals not at the level of individual patients, but at the level of all of the potential patients (total population) and has the internal resources to follow these goals.

It has also been given a new definition of health care:

> *Health care* is a way to organise life within the species, which aims to ensure its survival in the given environment and to provide the development in accordance with certain goals that used medicine as instrument as well as all social institutions that were developed in a given society.

It has been shown that a human is clearly preparing for artificial evolution; over time, the more and more he is separated from the habitat which gave rise him, and more and more is the creation of its own ecological niche. The subject of evolutionary changes are man's relationship with the environment; the means of evolution are the 'superstructures' and 'improvements' of its own body. It became clear that these improvements in the near future will completely change the way of life and ways of socialising of humanity.

It has been suggested that in the future the mankind will be divided on the basis of the whole set of attributes, leading to the gradual formation of its two branches:

> Long-living mankind with a high degree of readiness for the new and the desire for changes and 'milestone-modernised' body.

> Short-living mankind with a low degree of readiness for the new, fear of changes, and a sick, senile body.

It is clear that the long-living branch of humanity will be in the favourable evolutionary conditions and will soon be dominant.

We have seen that the history of medicine can actually be described as the history of the development of medical technologies, from the 'simulation', more like a religious rite, to not existing yet 'perfect' that will solve the specific medical problem of mankind at the root and for all.

It was also concluded that the medicine as a branch of scientific knowledge is still under the strong influence of religious tradition; it is highly lagging behind other exact sciences. The important reason for the backlog of medicine is the fact that its object of influence (human body) is protected by law; therefore, the experimental groundwork that uses other sciences in medicine is not applicable. Laws that describe the limits and scope of the activities of physicians and biologists (in contrast to other sciences) reflect the religious public morality of the past centuries and is constantly at odds with the current needs of the society and the possibilities of medical science.

The following definition of medical technology was given:

> *Medical technology* is a combination of knowledge, skills, techniques, and equipment that enable a qualified specialist to affect the natural development and changes in biological objects directly or indirectly, both individually and en masse, taking into account the reaction of the objects themselves and achieving goals with the greatest degree of probability. At a certain point, it becomes a tool for the health care system.

The simple arguments about the nature of the medical technologies have led us to an understanding of how the states for any reasons hopelessly lagging behind in medical technologies and training for medical personnel in today's globalised world face a tragic choice: of either being completely closed for the world and watch the slow decline of its population or allow developers of more effective medical technologies to control the quality and quantity of people on its territory.

To answer the question 'What are the products of medical technologies?' it has been shown that the product of medical technologies aimed at individual organism is changing the individual patient's body to preserve his life, eliminating pathological focus to the point of being comfortable, allowing him to work as well as showing some improvement in his body. The final products of the medical technologies aimed at a mass changes of organisms are an advantage over other individuals competing for a given economic or ecological niche.

Having examined the early health care systems, it becomes apparent that for any state there is a need to solve two interrelated global problems; they look very similar but have different targets:

> *First*, to provide an opportunity to conduct individual changes in the patient's body to preserve his life, elimination of pathological focus to the point of being comfortable, allowing him to work as well as show some improvement in his body at a reasonable price for him.

> *Second,* to get the opportunity to have an advantage over other groups of individuals competing for a economic or ecological niche, in terms of the nation state—to make the citizens of this state have a biological competitive advantage over citizens of other states (live longer and be more workable).

To answer the question 'Are there types of health care systems?' the answer was that at the moment the main criterion by which we can determine the type of HCS in general is exactly how well this system satisfies the above basic needs of the given society (from the first to the fifth point by Maslow). It was concluded that *at the given stage of development of the human society only one type of HCS can exist or there will be none.*

Next, the *general properties* of the health system were described:

- Statement of purpose
- Terms of goal
- Means to get the goal
- Tools for assessing the adequacy of the results
- Coverage of potential customers
- Price of the system's functioning to the public.

Analogy of the health system development was drawn with a phase transition known from thermodynamics, when the accumulation of the number of elements of the environment just simulates development, but does not lead to a new quality, which cannot occur without changes in the basic parameters of interaction of the system elements, a kind of social phase transition, in which all elements of the system having accumulated enough social energy at a time (by historical standards) change the state of the social environment throughout its volume by regularising it 'in a new way' and dramatically change the basic properties of the system, giving it the new opportunities for further quantitative growth, but at a new level.

Many analysts and futurists noted a tendency to weaken the control of the state; this process is most clearly visible in countries with post-industrial economy. Centres of real control in such society increasingly shifted to various public organisations which were both formal and informal and even temporary associations of citizens, including their full virtualisation. Against this background, there is an interesting question: What will happen with the health systems which are the flesh of the flesh of these moribund states, the expression of their state philosophy? Where will the centres of decision-making in the health systems of these areas move (it is already difficult to call them countries)?

In Section 3.A, we were told that if we consider the current strategic motives of the health care provider, government, and patient, we get the inevitable conclusion that these motives actually are economic; that is, the benefits of market players are defined. In the next stage of development of humanity, we will be ready to move from the economic to the humanistic goal-setting in health care, but previously we'll have to clarify this concept. Rather, the refinement of this concept will have to be done often in the future with the development of society. Social guarantees of the state, which in the developed countries now sound like 'I'll compensate your expenses for overcoming any medical and social problems, provided that you are a citizen of this state', will be translated into the biological plane, namely, that anyone belonging to the species Homo sapiens will be the subject of the guarantees of health and social care taken at the current level of technology, but the question of the availability of resources will be relegated to the background. Thus, the health systems will move to the biological guarantees of help for their population.

As the modern society is increasingly acquiring the features of the network community, the health system will have to be transformed in the same direction. It'll be controlled as an online community of patients, and patients will be considered by definition all members of the society. A significant part of the management of grassroots tasks have to be delegated to the patients, as well as to their cumulative total processing power, which will produce a preliminary analysis of medical data. This approach will help to get away from the control processes and start to manage the results, not only narrow medical ones but also to a large extent the social ones to the extent that they depend on the medical.

Big changes will occur in the concept of competition in medicine. The public opinion is starting movement towards a much greater social responsibility of medicine in general; the fact is that the population has begun to influence the clannish medical community, not so much in order to control 'what?' doctors make, but for the fact that people could make physicians also implement 'why?' and 'what for?', which in the immediate interests of doctors are not yet included. The means of competition is relevant, offering services that are the most appropriate to customers' expectations at a reasonable price. M. Porter says that this competition is counterproductive, because it offers a process, not an outcome for the patient. It seems to me that the root of the problem is that the patient and medical provider traditionally understood by the proposed product are *two different things*:

> Medical services provider while speaking about treatment is referring to the chain of process steps, reaching the best possible results for some time and known money.

> The patient under treatment is referring to the elimination of his medical and social problems to restore his ability to work within a certain time and fit in the available amount for him.

In the next few decades, the main efforts in medical management will be made to ensure that both the patient and health care provider understand the medical product as the same thing. That is, the main object of the struggle for quality of health care services will be information policy in relation to the patient. Society must stop lying to the patient about mythical achievements of medicine, but just keep informing him about the actual results achieved by the use of each medical technology. Public sources of information on the results of medical technologies that they can be trust should be made available. The patient now will begin to understand terms such as 'reliability and reproducibility of the medical outcome', 'accessibility of medical technology', 'the cost of supporting the medical outcome', 'medical outsourcing', and other terms, which are part of the practice among health care marketers for now.

Health care production has begun to build an integrated production chains of medical services, connecting the medical technologies in the most efficient manner. Those countries that have begun to use new technologies not just of medicine but also integrated chains of various medical and social technologies into one meaningful whole have abruptly pulled ahead in terms of providing additional value to their patients, namely, the stable quality of medical services chain, ending in the best possible results.

The market of health and social services will be mature and be divided into sectors within each medical specialty. The division will be based on medical conditions which are most suitable for organisations of full cycle business processes with quality control to deal with the probabilistic nature of the medical services results. At a certain stage of development of such a market, a new kind of competition for the new critical indicator will arise—extra years of life patients and their more numerous progeny.

In the near future, a person's life will be gradually transformed into a *continuous medical procedure*, which may not be seen in patients, and the treatment and correction will be implemented not only for already diagnosed medical conditions but also for those that with a very high degree of probability occur in a latent state, but they cannot be accurately diagnosed by the current degree of sensitivity of diagnostic equipment, and sometimes even for those that with a high probability will develop in the near future for the given sex-age group of the population; that is,. mass disease prevention will be a real point of state social policy and its successors—social organisations of citizens.

One of the possible scenarios of the breakthrough medical technology that has been specified is the scenario of bionic prosthetics of lost limbs and organs and their individual functions. Over time, this technology could enable the move to create fundamentally new organs that people would require under certain circumstances, due some professional needs or living in special environments. Also, it could be applied to improve the communication capabilities of initially healthy people, creating new ways of socialisation of the population, the acquisition of new work skills, and the emergence of fundamentally new jobs and new careers. Prosthetics can completely change the face of preventive medicine in the near future; in particular, it may be possible to change the properties of human organs and systems so that age-related failures do not occur at all or occur at a much later age.

In Section 4.B, the question about the danger of turning the patient into an object of patent protection because of the mass of bionic devices in his body and also because of the possible aesthetic and artistic manipulations of his appearance was raised. It was pointed that the ways out of this situation are only two: either to create a government's financial structure, which would carry out all the payments on behalf of the citizens with prosthesis, or to limit the patent right, completely eliminating from it all biological objects.

Further, in Section 4.B, it was predicted that in the near future all the citizens of the state will be considered as patients, by definition. In such circumstances, the state for diagnostic activity will no longer need formal permission. This transition is the most important change in the paradigm of the medical officer, from the earliest times. In this case, the health care system leads to the concept of continuous monitoring of all the citizens-patients. Namely, this concept allows one to realise the dream of preventive medicine that cannot be reliably applied on the technological stage of subjective and instrumental medical examinations. There will be a gradual transition to the creation of a universal friendly-living environment, which keeps track of all beings in it who are the members of the species Homo sapiens.

In the pharmaceutical industry, a gradual abandonment of the concept of mass production of finished products 'for all' in favour of the concept of the production of personalised medicines for narrow target groups of patients can occur, as well as the production of 'pharmaceutical intermediates,' designed to finishing in specialised pharmacies. The scheme of relations between the physician and the pharmacist can go back to a medieval version, where a doctor would write a prescription for the pharmacist, who would prepare an individual drug for the individual patient.

In Section 4.D, it was said that in the future the technology of cultivation of the individual organs can be developed. If this technology is implemented, then at some point it may be worth less than the traditional treatment of the patient's organ. In this case, curative technologies very quickly, within a generation of doctors, will be left as economically inefficient and will be replaced by technology of driven regeneration of organs.

With the technology of bionic prosthetic organs and their individual features, people will soon be born having already been adapted to living in an environment specially created for them. What exactly are these habitats we cannot know in advance; it will be solved by the residents themselves: It is possible that originally the difference in air pressure, atmospheric composition, temperature and humidity, the presence of various types of radiation, etc. will be discussed.

In Section 4.G, it was concluded that humanity is becoming more diverse in terms of health. It points to the situation where the percentage of the population that can be officially recognised as healthy all the time is reduced, which gives the population a clear but false impression that the doctors and the health system as a whole are getting worse and worse in coping with their work. Thus, it will proceed to the artificial diversity of the human population, which will mark a new stage in its evolutionary development. Unlike earlier, this stage will be completely man-made. At some stage, *different types of human organisms* will appear.

It has been said that, namely, the work of the state to find a balance between all the participants in health and social processes leads to a fundamentally new branch of law, which was not in the classical Roman law or in the Civil Code of Napoleon. This section describes the rules by which the given society reached an agreement to control its quantity, longevity, and level of health. The human society in its history did not experience such needs before. Changes in this legislation can lead to completely separate types of medical care and, accordingly, based on them the separate health systems designed for specific types of human organisms.

In Section 5.A, it was said that in the near future the merger of several medical specialties is inevitable: endocrinology, neurology, cytology, immunology, and medical genetics, and some others in one super-specialty which will be concerned with the issues of internal control terrestrial organisms in general and in particular the human body, as well as issues of information interchange between these organisms. So far, I suggest naming this science biocybernetics, and in that, the part of it which will cover the human body should be called medical biocybernetics. Such an external control system which allows one to correct the state of human and, moreover, to rebuild his body structure is actually the next evolutionary step in the development of the species, the universal tool for changing himself. The tools can bring about total changes in the internal structure and appearance of the human body, and also in creating human organs which could not (or not yet) emerge in the logic of the evolutionary process.

In Section 5.B, it was suggested that in the near future *consumer explosion in the new market of body changes* can happen. These changes and superstructures of body as well as the nervous system will lead to a lengthening of the human life, which, in turn, will cause the changes in the mentality of the average man, his attitude towards himself, his health, and his offspring. Along with the increase in the lifespan, changes in the economy of mankind will happen, which is tied to the life expectancy of human, which is much more than one might think.

In Section 5.D, the impact of the rapid extension of the average life expectancy (ALE) was considered; it was said that careless and widespread use of such technologies without any preparation of the economy and the social structures of society can cause a domino effect, completely redrawing the entire economy of mankind and all the social and financial airbags of our modern society caving in. Before the application of biomedical technologies, which are significantly extending the life of humanity as a whole, the consequences for next generations must be carefully calculated and, if necessary, the structure of society and the dominant mode of production adjusted beforehand. A special challenge will consist of the fact that these calculations and corrections for now will have to be performed on a *global scale*, for the planet as a whole.

In Section 5.G, it was predicted that processes of transformation in the medical profession will logically lead to the situation where the *medical profession would be 'dissolved' in the population*; that is, every able-bodied person would have the credentials to diagnose and treat a certain spectrum of diseases characterised by a low price of error. The significant part of today's activity of physicians is that, namely, diagnostic activity is leaving the doctor's hands and going into the hands of the clients. Public opinion has gradually moved to the concept that doing small repairs of his own body is the duty of the citizen and that the inability to do so is a sign of backwardness and lack of education.

Index

A

abnormalities   12, 58
abortion   162-3, 193
adaptability   43, 49
adaptability, degree of   43
adaptation   33, 46, 220, 257-9
age cohorts   150, 152, 154-5, 205, 207, 292-3
ALE (average life expectancy)   41-3, 46, 48, 154, 215, 217, 233, 293, 319
anatomists   278
Anthropology   283
Aurelius, Marcus   20

B

baby boom   147
behaviour   34, 170, 260-1, 278-9
Beveridge   86-7, 89
biological objects   10, 32, 66, 70, 78, 120, 129, 131, 225, 229, 241, 265, 267, 310, 316
biologists   69, 120, 156, 310
bionics   224-6, 285
Bismarck, Otto von   86-7, 89
brain   34, 218, 221, 233, 278-82, 304
breeding, selective   13, 15, 18, 25, 50, 308

C

care cycles   182
cells   30-1, 273-4
Civil Code of Napoleon   318
Collective value system   96
competition   63, 81, 132, 138, 164, 167-72, 174-5, 177, 180-1, 183, 187-8, 211, 221, 313-15
Cro-Magnon   32, 34, 41

D

Darwin, Charles   18, 33, 66
dead medical technology   77
demographic problems   141-2, 154, 160
demographic pyramid   144-5, 153-4, 157-8, 292
demographic transition   148, 154, 157, 211, 292
depopulation   150, 154, 157
disabilities   38, 87, 127, 226, 248-51, 253, 264
diseases   14, 26, 37, 57, 60-1, 78-9, 84, 87, 94, 112, 116, 130, 160, 171, 178, 198, 208-9, 219, 221, 228, 230-1, 245, 249-50, 253, 270-1, 275, 296
chronic   92, 290, 293-4
heart   300
infectious   36-7, 83, 87, 94, 148
doctor-patient relationship   261

T

www.ingramcontent.com/pod-product-compliance
Lightning Source LLC
Chambersburg PA
CBHW030419290526
45786CB00001B/53